KNACK®
MAKE IT EASY

# PREGNANCY GUIDE

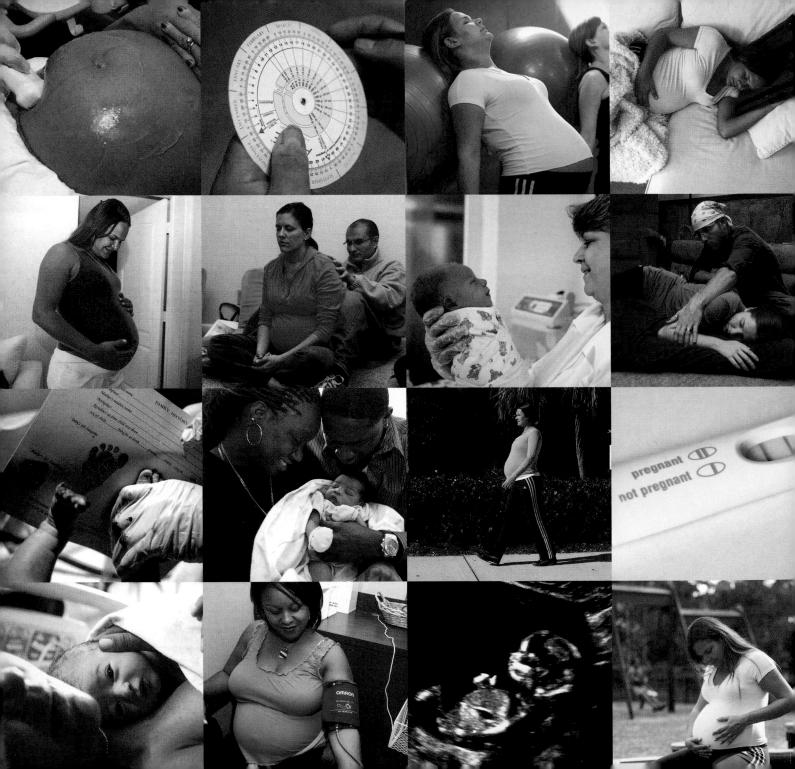

KNACK®

# PREGNANCY GUIDE

An Illustrated Handbook for Every Trimester

**Brenda J. Lane, LCCE, CD(DONA), and Ilana T. Kirsch, M.D., FACOG**

**Photographs by Carline Jean**

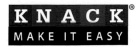

*Guilford, Connecticut*
An imprint of The Globe Pequot Press

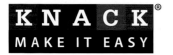

**KNACK**®
MAKE IT EASY

Copyright © 2009 by Morris Book Publishing, LLC

Editor-in-Chief: Maureen Graney
Editor: Katie Benoit
Cover Design: Paul Beatrice, Bret Kerr
Text Design: Paul Beatrice
Layout: Joanna Beyer
Cover and Back Cover Photos by Carline Jean
Illustrations by Robert L. Prince
Interior photos by Carline Jean with the exception of p. xii (left): Vivid Pixels/shutterstock; p. xii (right): szefei/shutterstock; p. 1 (left): Suzanne Tucker/shutterstock; p. 1 (right): Vivid Pixels/shutterstock; p. 3 (left): © istockphoto; p. 15 (right): Jacek Chabraszewski/shutterstock; p. 16 (right): © istockphoto; p. 17 (left): © istockphoto; p. 17 (right): © istockphoto; p. 20 (right): © Riverlim | Dreamstime.com; p. 23 (right): © istockphoto; p. 35 (left): Tobik/shutterstock; p. 40 (right): © istockphoto; p. 50 (right): Monkey Business Images/shutterstock; p. 51 (right): iofoto/shutterstock; p. 52 (right): © istockphoto; p. 54 (right): © istockphoto; p. 55 (right): Sophie Louise Asselin/shutterstock; p. 58 (left): Petrenko Andriy/shutterstock; p. 58 (right): Monkey Business Images/shutterstock; p. 59 (right): Simone van den Berg/shutterstock; p. 63 (left): © istockphoto; p. 64 (right): © Iofoto | Dreamstime.com; p. 65 (left): © istockphoto; p. 68 (right): © istockphoto; p. 73 (right): © istockphoto; p. 74 (right): © istockphoto; p. 78 (right): © istockphoto; p. 80 (right): Tiplyashin Anatoly/shutterstock; p. 85 (right): Ken Hurst/shutterstock; p. 88 (right): © Alwekelo | Dreamstime.com; p. 95 (left): © Iofoto | Dreamstime.com; p. 97 (left): © Elemi | Dreamstime.com; p. 100 (right): © Monkeybusiness | Dreamstime.com; p. 108 (right): © Erdosain | Dreamstime.com; p. 110 (right): Vincek/shutterstock; p. 116 (right): © istockphoto; p. 117 (left): © istockphoto; p. 118 (right): © istockphoto; p. 119 (left): © Ngothyeaun | Dreamstime.com; p. 134 (right): Kim Ruoff/shutterstock; p. 135 (right): Galina Barskaya/shutterstock; p. 138 (right): © istockphoto; p. 139 (left): © istockphoto; p. 141 (right): © istockphoto; p. 143 (left): © istockphoto; p. 145 (left): © Johncarlet... | Dreamstime.com; p. 162 (right): © Arielmarti... | Dreamstime.com; p. 163 (left): © istockphoto; p. 164 (right): Monkey Business Images/shutterstock; p. 165 (left): © Gonzalomed... | Dreamstime.com; p. 166 (right): © Jupiter Images; p. 167 (left): © Bradcalkin... | Dreamstime.com; p. 170 (right): Vivid Pixels/shutterstock; p. 176 (right): © Madja | Dreamstime.com; p. 177 (left): Dean Mitchell/shutterstock; p. 177 (right): © Monkeybusiness | Dreamstime.com; p. 180 (right Monkey Business Images/shutterstock; p. 181 (right): Monkey Business Images/shutterstock; p. 183 (right): © istockphoto; p. 191 (left): Joel Blit/shutterstock; p. 191 (right): Galina Barskaya/shutterstock; p. 195 (left): © Vladacanon | Dreamstime.com; p. 197 (left): © Chiyacat | Dreamstime.com; p. 218 (right): © Alangh | Dreamstime.com; p. 226 (right): Zsolt Nyulaszi/shutterstock

Library of Congress Cataloging-in-Publication Data is available on file.
ISBN 978-1-59921-512-9

The following manufacturers/names appearing in *Knack Pregnancy Guide* are trademarks:
BirthWorks©, BlackBerry®, Bradley Method®, Dura*Kold®, Gatorade®, HypnoBirthing®, Jell-O®, KY®, NutraSweet®, OxyContin®, Percocet®, Scotchgard™, Splenda®

Printed in China
10 9 8 7 6 5 4 3 2 1

I am grateful for the opportunity to use my God-given gifts in supporting many families in the last 18 years. Many thanks also go to Barb Doyen, my agent, for her encouragement during the challenges of writing this book. I am indebted to my husband Chris and daughters, Carly and Alyson, for their daily support. Finally I wish to thank my best cheerleader, Jill, for the blessing of her friendship.

—Brenda Lane

To all of the moms and moms-to-be.

—Carline Jean

# CONTENTS

# INTRODUCTION

One thing you can say for certain about pregnancy is that everyone will have an opinion to share with you, whether you ask for it or not. Pregnancy seems to go hand in hand with very strong attitudes about the "right" things to eat, the "right" class to take for childbirth, the "right" way to have your baby, and so on. The truth is that there are many valid choices with regard to pregnancy that are available to women today. Some choices are proven by research or scientific fact to be safer or healthier for mother or baby, such as the choice to breastfeed. Some are just good common sense, such as eating more natural or organic foods rather than a diet full of processed, ready-made foods. And other choices are personal opinions that folks feel passionately about, such as whether or not to undergo prenatal testing.

## A mother's decision making takes into account her own personal history and information gathering during pregnancy.

When you are planning your own pregnancy or in the early weeks of pregnancy, you will soon recognize that it takes time to develop your own philosophy. You might hear a friend recommend a certain care provider, but you know that you will need to meet with the provider yourself and ask him a number of questions that are important to you. You will have your own medical history, your own set of ideas, and even your own worries that weigh heavily into all of your decision making. None of these decisions relating to pregnancy are made overnight. Making choices requires reading, research, and information gathering from numerous sources. Some of these sources may include the Internet, books, magazines, medical journals, medical care providers, childbirth educators, doulas, friends, and family. In fact, so much can influence you during your journey that you may end up with a whole different set of ideas at the end of nine months than what you started with! It is also quite common for mothers to change their minds about their choices from one pregnancy to the next.

Despite the avalanche of information today's expectant couples have at their fingertips, myths and outdated advice about the childbearing year abound. This is one reason why this book includes the latest research on pregnancy, as well as numerous references in our directory at the back of the book. When you are doing your own research, bear in mind that guidelines are constantly being updated so by the time you have your next baby, some of the former advice may have changed. A perfect example of this can be seen in the new weight-gain recommendation for mothers. Only a few years ago, moms were told to gain roughly twenty-five to thirty-five pounds during pregnancy, allowing more if you were underweight or less if you were overweight at the start of your pregnancy. Now the recommended weight gain is much more precise and is based on the mother's own BMI (body mass index).

## Writing a birth plan during pregnancy can help the mother to communicate her choices to her birth team before going into labor.

Expectant parents can take an active role in every decision along the way, rather than being bystanders. If you think that you need not seek any information beyond talking to your care provider, think again. No single care provider has all of the answers to every question you will have. Not to mention, as caring and supportive as they may be, your doctor or midwife will have her own personal biases and histories that influence her particular philosophies. You might begin to think of your care provider as a consultant, if you will, in your pregnancy. His expert opinion will be invaluable to you,

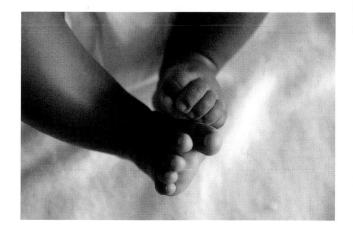

especially if complications occur. But many of the choices are still yours to make.

One of the ways that you can organize your preferences and decisions about birth most effectively is by writing a birth plan. While a written birth plan doesn't work for all mothers, it can provide valuable information for your birth team. Be sure you research your plan through talking with your care provider, reading up with reputable sources, and avoiding copying generic birth plans directly off the Internet.

You certainly wouldn't buy a new car without considering your budget, the features you are looking for, and financing. Nor would you plan a wedding without carefully orchestrating all of the details from the invitations to cutting the cake and everything in between. Having a baby ranks even higher on the scale of life's most precious moments, so why would you not take great care in thinking about what is most important to you? Just as unexpected events happen at weddings or you end up with a car that is different than the one you intended to buy, labor and birth can also be unpredictable. Just because you may need to alter a few things along the way during birth does not mean parents should leave all their choices up to someone else. Not to mention that trying to make decisions that you know nothing about during the throes of labor contractions will be next to impossible.

## Staying on top of all of your new responsibilities can be challenging for today's busy parents.

The couples we have highlighted in this book are giving you an inside view to some of the choices they are making with regard to pregnancy and planning for birth. Some of the couples are making choices to use a midwife and give birth at a birth center. Others are planning to use an epidural in a hospital setting. Some plan to breastfeed for as long as possible. A few are returning to their careers after maternity leave, while the others are staying at home. This is the perfect illustration that many choices are valid and each couple has taken the time to find the ones that best suit them.

Just like you, these future parents are recognizing that their many other responsibilities do not stop the moment they become pregnant. The new demands of pregnancy must somehow fit into your already busy routine of working, doing errands, paying bills, spending time with friends and family, and maintaining a home. Your head can spin with everything you need to accomplish in just nine short months. With this in mind, our book has many tips to make your months of pregnancy easier, such as using a slow cooker for healthy meal planning, help in planning your baby shower, baby-proofing your home, and "to do" checklists for each trimester of pregnancy to keep you organized.

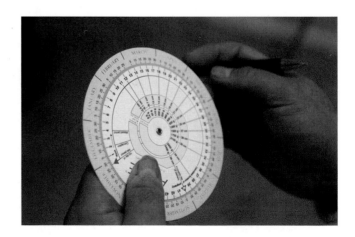

## Pregnancy and childbirth bring both challenges and joyous moments to mothers- and fathers-to-be.

Mothers often share that one of the most exciting things about pregnancy is being able to hear the baby's heartbeat and see their baby on an ultrasound. We have included a month-by-month look at your baby's development as well as a description of all of the miraculous changes taking place throughout the entire nine months. Your baby's health depends on your good eating habits. This is one reason why we have two chapters dedicated to the vital topic of nutrition during pregnancy. Since eating well is more and more challenging to today's busy moms, we have tips on healthy snacks when you have no time or appetite for big meals. In addition, there are reminders in our trimester sections to make certain you are getting those extra nutrients when your baby needs them most.

Undoubtedly one of the most challenging aspects of pregnancy for many women is morning sickness. If you are one of the 80 to 90 percent of mothers who have nausea and/or vomiting at any point during your day, you will be relieved to find an extensive list of helpful tips for managing those symptoms. Beyond eating saltine crackers, our first-trimester section includes some of the newest methods that can help mothers cope when they may have weeks or months of feeling sick.

By the time you work through the many weeks of morning sickness, the aches and pains of your growing baby taking up more and more space, and all of your preparations for birth and parenting, you may suddenly realize that your life is about to change all over again when you become a mother. Just remember that all of the new life skills that both of you have acquired during pregnancy, such as researching your options, connecting with trusted people in your life, and asking for help when you need it, will prepare you for life's next chapter ahead. Thank you for allowing us to share this nine-month journey with you!

# GETTING STARTED
## Your physical and emotional health is vital as you prepare for your pregnancy

Your journey is just beginning. As you prepare for your upcoming pregnancy, here are a few things to help make your journey a bit easier.

One of the most crucial aspects of a healthy pregnancy is nutrition. Even if you are not yet pregnant, you can get off to a good start by eating nutritious, vitamin-packed foods that include plenty of folic acid. Why is such a big deal made about folic acid? Because studies show that getting 400 micrograms a day of this B vitamin before pregnancy may help prevent neural tube defects, a class of birth defect including spina bifida. Your baby will thank you for providing him/her with all of those great nutrients.

### Healthy Mothers

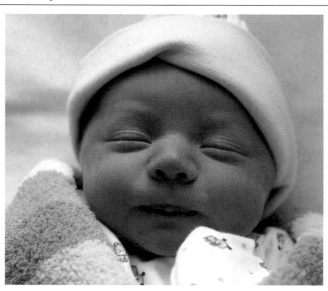

- Even before pregnancy is the best time to start taking good care of you!

- Remember to communicate to your partner, friends, and family about what you need before, during, and after pregnancy.

- Find times during your busy schedule for relaxation and reflection just because.

- Think about all of the things that make you happy and make them happen.

### Healthy Fathers

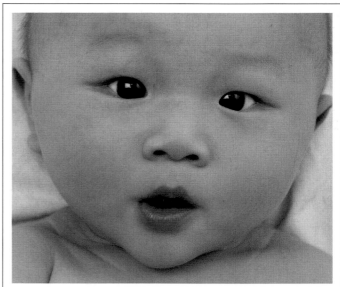

- Your life is about to change, so get ready.

- You will never have all the answers, but sharing with another dad can ease your worries.

- This is great time to think about how you view your role and the kind of father you want to be.

- Spending more time with your wife and future baby is one of the best ways to show that you love them.

Pre-pregnancy is the best time to begin the process of decision making regarding motherhood. Will you work outside the home? Can you stay at home with your baby? Would you prefer part-time or full-time work? You may not come up with all of the answers now, but exploring what is important to you in the months before conception is ideal.

Do not neglect your emotional well-being as you prepare to have a baby. Do you feel confident in becoming a mother? Journaling can help you get in touch with your emotions about pregnancy and motherhood.

**ZOOM**

Journal Questions
What are my biggest concerns about becoming a mother? What are ways that I cope with stress or uncertainty? How is my relationship with my family? What are my goals before baby arrives? Where can I find support?

## Healthy Pregnancy

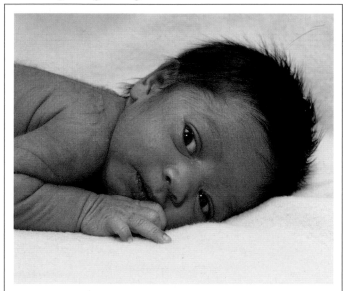

- Mom and baby need even more sleep, since their bodies are going through great changes.

- What mom eats, baby gets, so feed baby well!

- Pregnancy can be nearly stress-free if mothers can stay organized and feel supported.

- Take time to stop and enjoy the amazing changes during each month of pregnancy.

## Healthy Babies

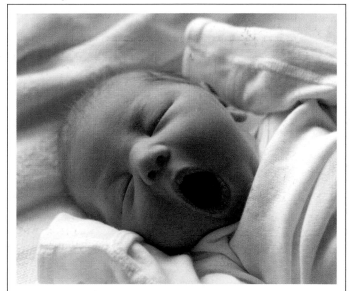

- Your baby is aware of life outside the uterus well before he/she is born.

- You and your baby have an ongoing exchange of nutrients and hormones throughout your entire pregnancy.

- Bonding with your baby may start from the very first kick or a first glimpse at the baby's ultrasound.

- Raising your baby starts with making wise decisions during your pregnancy.

# MAKING ROOM FOR BABY

## Parents need to evaluate their living space as well as their finances before pregnancy

The optimal time to make room for your baby is before you are pregnant or during the early stages of pregnancy, so that you have plenty of time to settle in. Parents may decide to buy larger homes, add on a room or two, or re-design their existing living space during pregnancy to make more room for the baby. Using the space you already have is a lot less expensive than adding on rooms or buying a larger home. Part of your planning should include organizing a timetable with any projects that need to be done as well as estimated costs for any renovations that you might need to do.

What about the actual costs involved in having a baby? Experts agree that it can cost as much as $150,000 to raise

### Estimated Costs to Have a Baby

- Crib: $200–$1,200
- Stroller: $100–$150
- Changing Table: $130–$500
- Layette (including clothing and linens): $100–$300
- Diapers: $500–$800 per year
- Formula: $100 and up per month (breastfeeding saves money)
- Vaginal birth: $6,000–$8,000
- Cesarean: $10,000–$12,000
- (Insurance should cover most of the above birth-related expenses. Using a midwife or birth center can lower these costs.)

*Tight Squeezes*

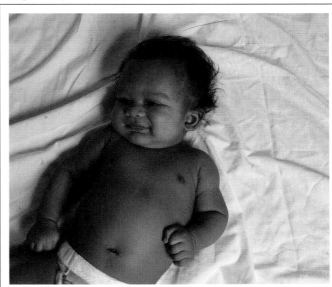

- The baby does not take up much room, but all of those baby items seem to take over what space you do have.

- The good thing is that some parents find that they do not need to have a separate bedroom or nursery until their baby is older.

- If space is tight, you may be able to put a crib and dresser in your guest room or office rather than converting an entire room for the baby's nursery.

- Plus, your baby may be in your room at night for the first few weeks to make late-night feedings easier!

a child until the age of 18. In the first year of life alone, baby expenses can reach as high as $7,000 or more. Adding health-care expenses to that figure can be daunting. However, there are ways to save on baby items by borrowing them or finding deals at yard sales or gently used items online. You can also save hundreds of dollars in the first year by breastfeeding versus feeding your baby formula.

## GREEN●LIGHT

You may be interested in finding baby items that are organic or eco-friendly. Some products may be made from recycled materials. Look for companies that offer baby clothing, for example, made with natural fibers and fewer chemicals. Or look for baby furniture that is non-toxic and constructed with natural materials.

### Borrowing Baby Items

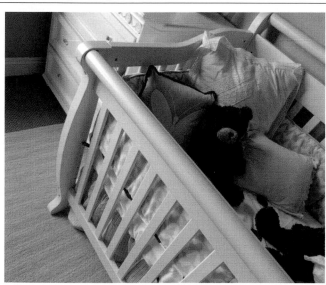

- Talk to your friends or family who have recently had a baby to see what baby items they can let you borrow.

- You might save hundreds of dollars by borrowing some of the more expensive baby items, such as cribs, changing tables, strollers, and high chairs.

- If they are good quality, many of these baby items hold up well enough to last through several years of use.

- Make sure you ask if they want the items back or if you should pass them on to another family.

### Save Now for College

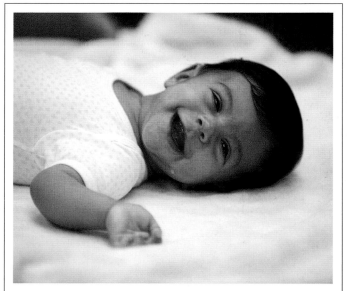

- It may seem like college is very far in your future. However, with college expenses skyrocketing, you can benefit from saving as early as possible.

- There are many college savings plans that are available to parents today.

- Some plans will allow you to have a designated amount of money taken out of your paycheck.

- Financial advisors should be able to help you find a plan that falls within your budget.

# UNDERSTANDING YOUR FERTILITY

## Eating a healthy diet may help mothers increase their chances of conception

For some women, getting pregnant will be very easy. Others find that trying to conceive takes longer than they expected. About one-quarter of all women will have difficulty becoming pregnant.

The best time for you to become pregnant is right around ovulation. Most women ovulate about eleven to sixteen days after the first day of their last menstrual period. Your ovary will release an egg, which travels into your fallopian tube before it is met by your partner's sperm. Following ejaculation, about 240 million to 360 million sperm enter the mother's vagina. But of course, it only takes one of these tiny sperm to fertilize the egg. The additional lubrication you experience during

### Ovulation

Most mothers ovulate about two weeks after the first day of their last menstrual period.

Your most fertile time is within a few days surrounding the time of ovulation, or about twelve to sixteen days after the first day of your last period.

If your cycles are longer, you may ovulate later in the month and if they are shorter than twenty-eight days, ovulation can occur sooner.

If you are having difficulty conceiving, it is a good idea to chart your cycles for several months, especially if you have never done so.

### Ovulation Kits

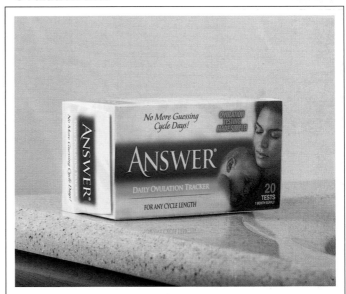

- Ovulation kits can be helpful if you do not have a regular menstrual cycle.

- You might consider trying a kit for only a month or two, since kits can be hard to use.

- Even though they are about 97 percent effective in detecting the LH hormone, ovulation kits cannot confirm that you are actually ovulating.

- Ovulation kits are available in grocery stores and pharmacies and cost between $15 and $50.

ovulation aids the speed at which the sperm can reach your egg. You can increase your chance of getting pregnant simply by making love every other day right around the time you expect ovulation to occur.

What gets in the way of fertility? Studies show that mothers who are overweight or underweight or mothers who smoke have a more difficult time conceiving than those who are at their normal weight. Ovulation kits make it easier for women to understand their body's monthly changes and can be a help for women who may have trouble getting pregnant.

## Romance

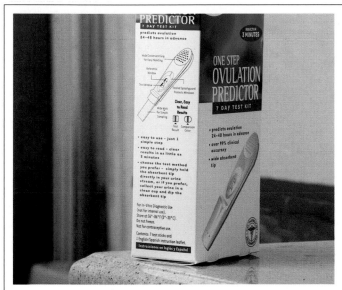

- Planning to conceive a baby shouldn't just be about the mechanics.

- Sometimes you can focus too much on the calendar, tests, and kits instead of sharing love with one another.

- If you know when you are ovulating, bring in some quiet music, candles, flowers, and romance to make it a beautiful event.

- Remember that spontaneity in your love-making throughout the month can be fun, too.

### Tips on Getting Pregnant

- Make love around the time you think you are ovulating.
- Use an ovulation kit.
- Eat a healthy diet.
- Lose weight if you are overweight.
- Gain weight if you are underweight.
- Reduce stress.
- Quit smoking.
- Reduce/limit alcohol consumption.

# USING MONTHLY CHARTS

## Charting your cycle is easier than ever with this list of monthly signs and symptoms

Tracking your monthly cycle can be an easy way to figure out when you are fertile and increase your chance of conception. Your monthly chart should include the date, the cycle day (number one is the first day you bleed), and your basal body temperature. It should also include comments on the quality of your cervical mucous and presence of other ovulation symptoms, such as ovary pain, cramping, bloating, and fluid retention.

First thing in the morning, take your basal body temperature (BBT) with a basal body thermometer and record it. This can be done either vaginally or orally, but use the same method consistently. Your BBT can be recorded as a graph so

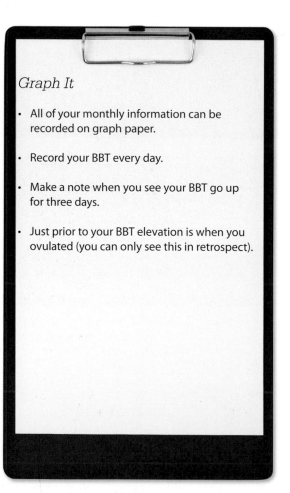

### Graph It

- All of your monthly information can be recorded on graph paper.

- Record your BBT every day.

- Make a note when you see your BBT go up for three days.

- Just prior to your BBT elevation is when you ovulated (you can only see this in retrospect).

### What to Include

- BBT temperatures on a graph

- Date

- Day in cycle

- Cervical mucous

- Ovulation results, signs, and symptoms

- Home pregnancy test (HPT) results

that during ovulation you will notice that your BBT will drop slightly. After ovulation, progesterone causes your temperature to increase approximately 0.6 degrees from what it was in the first half of your cycle. When your BBT has been elevated for three straight days, you can be certain that you ovulated right before the first day your temperature increased.

Other signs of ovulation include vaginal discharge (similar to the consistency of egg whites). About one-fifth of women also have sharp, knife-like pain during ovulation, known as mittelschmerz.

## Basal Thermometers

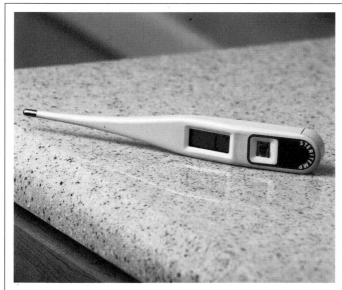

- There are a variety of basal thermometers that you can use to chart your BBT.

- One of the easiest types to use is a digital basal thermometer.

- Digital basal thermometers are very fast and only take about thirty to sixty seconds to read your temperature.

- Basal thermometers can record your body temperature within a range from 96 to 99.5 degrees.

## Basal Thermometers, continued

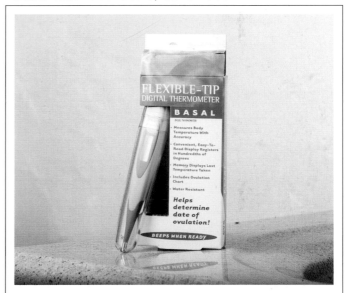

FLEXIBLE-TIP
DIGITAL THERMOMETER

**BASAL**

- Measures Body Temperature With Accuracy
- Convenient, Easy-To-Read Display Registers in Hundredths of Degrees
- Memory Displays Last Temperature Taken
- Includes Ovulation Chart
- Water Resistant

**Helps determine date of ovulation!**

BEEPS WHEN READY

- Basal thermometers have the advantage of accuracy within one one-hundredth of a degree.

- In order to improve the accuracy of your BBT recording, be sure to take your temperature after five hours of continuous sleep.

- You can find a BBT thermometer at most department stores or pharmacies.

- The cost for a BBT thermometer typically runs about $10.

# CONFIRMING THE HUNCH

## If you take a home pregnancy test too soon, your results may not be accurate

While a few mothers may know immediately after conception that they are pregnant, most do not. Early symptoms of pregnancy are not the same for every woman, so getting confirmation with a pregnancy test can put your mind at ease.

Home pregnancy tests (HPTs) are available in most grocery stores and pharmacies and are a convenient way to confirm your pregnancy. You can test your first morning urine as early as the first day of your missed period. HPTs have a 90 percent accuracy rate the first day your period is late and a 97 percent accuracy rate when your period is one week late.

The HPT detects the level of human chorionic gonadotropin (hCG) in the mother's urine. HCG is a hormone produced

### Am I Pregnant?

- Feeling bloated or a sense of fullness
- Slight sensation of cramping
- Breast tenderness
- Frequent urination
- Missed period
- Fatigue
- Lighter than normal period

### Tips on Taking HPTs

- Take seven to ten days after missed period
- Use first morning urine
- Check expiration date on package
- Follow instructions in box

by your placenta and can be detected in your blood or urine from eight to twelve days after conception. If you are having symptoms of early pregnancy and need an earlier test result than what is available with an HPT, you can visit a local pregnancy clinic or your care provider's office to have a blood test. Blood tests can detect even smaller amounts of hCG a few days earlier than in the mother's urine. Sometimes your care provider will want to repeat your blood test in a few days to make sure the levels of hCG are increasing.

**ZOOM**

HCG plays a huge role in early pregnancy by helping in the secretion of progesterone, preparing the lining of the uterus, helping to stimulate estrogen, and assisting in the development of the placenta.

## *Home Pregnancy Test*

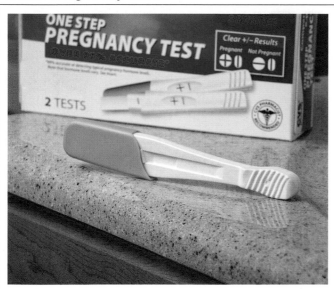

- Most HPTs require that you urinate across the stick provided.

- Some HPTs ask that you collect your urine in a cup and then dip the stick into it.

- Most tests ask you wait about five minutes before checking the result.

- If a line or a plus symbol appears—even if it's faint— it is positive, meaning you're pregnant.

## *Test Results*

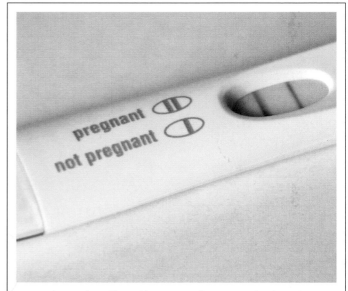

- Results can be affected by taking the HPT before you miss your period.

- Not all mothers produce the same amount of HCG early in the pregnancy.

- If you are taking medications for infertility, they can affect the accuracy of test results.

- Prescription and over-the-counter medications should not affect your HPT result.

# HEY BABY—CONCEPTION
## Calculating your baby's expected date of arrival is simple, even if you're not sure when you conceived

Congratulations! You are now pregnant. As soon as you get the positive test result on a blood test or your HPT, you can calculate your baby's expected date of arrival, also known as your "due date."

Some mothers will know the exact date of conception. If you do, then one way to calculate your due date is to count thirty-eight weeks from that date. For example, if you know the baby was conceived on May 15, your baby's due date is approximately February 6 of the following year.

You can also figure out your due date based on your last menstrual period. Using this formula, known as Naegele's rule, take the first date of your last menstrual period (LMP), subtract

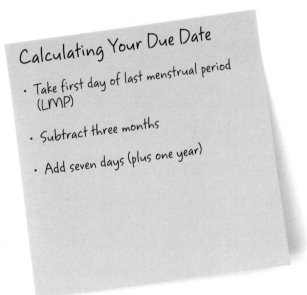

**Calculating Your Due Date**

- Take first day of last menstrual period (LMP)

- Subtract three months

- Add seven days (plus one year)

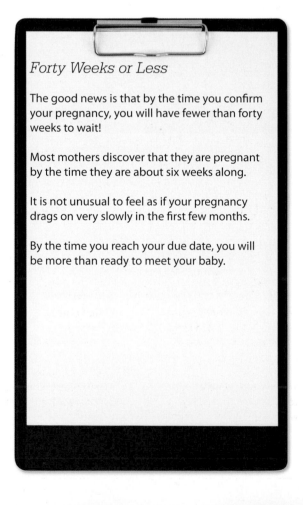

*Forty Weeks or Less*

The good news is that by the time you confirm your pregnancy, you will have fewer than forty weeks to wait!

Most mothers discover that they are pregnant by the time they are about six weeks along.

It is not unusual to feel as if your pregnancy drags on very slowly in the first few months.

By the time you reach your due date, you will be more than ready to meet your baby.

three months from it and add seven days plus one year. So if the first day of your LMP was May 20, you would subtract three months (which would give us February 20), then add seven days (which brings us to February 27), and then add one year. So your estimated due date is February 27.

So now that your pregnancy test is confirmed and you know your due date, congratulations on discovering that you will become a mother in just a few months! This is the beginning of an amazing journey, so hang on and join us for the rest of your ride!

**ZOOM**

Rather than a magical date, remember that your baby is most likely to arrive within a two-week period before or after your due date. Eighty percent of mothers give birth within one week before or after their due date. This means that 20 percent of mothers will give birth more than seven days early or seven days past their due date.

## Lunar Months

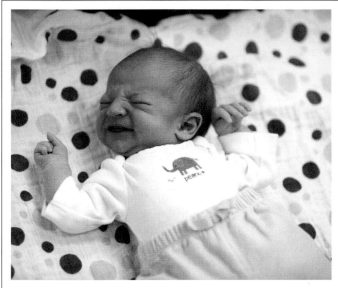

- Each lunar month is actually twenty-eight days in length (comprised of four weeks of seven days).

- You can also see that your total pregnancy is forty weeks or 280 days in length.

- How that translates is that your pregnancy is a total of ten lunar months long.

- But just remember that your baby can't read a calendar so he will arrive when he is ready.

## Help Needed

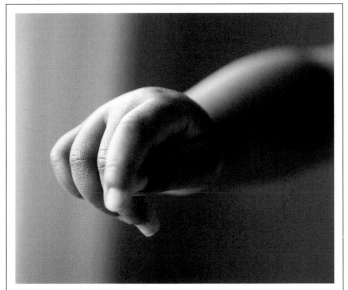

- What if you can't remember when you conceived or the first day of your LMP?

- Or what if your cycle is so irregular that you don't know when you might have gotten pregnant?

- Your care provider can look at other things like examining the size of your uterus or listening to your baby's heartbeat to estimate your baby's due date.

- You can also have an ultrasound to help determine your estimated due date.

# EATING FOR TWO

## Check out our twenty-four best pregnancy foods and fun ways to include them in your diet

A healthy diet is not only great for your baby but also for you. Here are our top twenty-four favorite pregnancy foods. They are jam-packed with vitamins, rich in flavor, and generally easy on your wallet.

Vegetables: broccoli, sweet potatoes, spinach, tomatoes, Swiss chard, romaine lettuce. Fruits: bananas, blueberries, cantaloupe, papaya, raspberries, prunes. Grains and legumes: whole-grain wheat, bran flakes, lentils, black or red beans. Fish and meat: salmon, halibut, chicken, lean beef. Dairy: eggs, low-fat yogurt, skim milk. Nuts: almonds, cashews.

One way to enjoy a variety of foods is to try pairings of different foods. You might even think of "eating for two" as eating

KNACK PREGNANCY GUIDE

### Raspberries and Yogurt

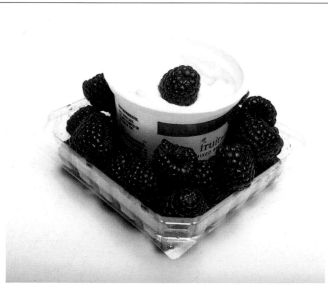

- This combo of fruit and a dairy is a favorite for breakfast or a snack.

- You get plenty of calcium and protein in the yogurt.

- Don't forget that milk products such as yogurt contain an important vitamin for pregnancy—vitamin B12.

- Raspberries have tons of vitamin C and eight grams of fiber in each serving.

### Romaine Lettuce with Tomatoes

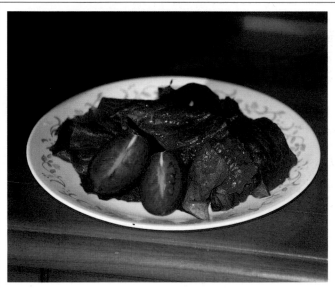

- Romaine lettuce and tomatoes are the start of a tasty salad that you can add to lunch or dinner or are fine to eat as is. Romaine lettuce provides vitamins A, C, K, and potassium and is loaded with good antioxidants to reduce cholesterol.

- Tomatoes are a good source of several vitamins, including A, C, and K.

- Don't forget to get your dressing on the side since piling on the dressing can add way too much fat and calories.

one healthy food item for you and another one for your baby.

Try pairing a carb with a protein. Or you could pair two fruits or vegetables with different textures or colors together. Your meal or snack should look like an artist's palette, mixing varieties of colors together! Remember that the more colorful your plate is with assorted proteins, carbohydrates, fruits, and vegetables, the better it is for you and baby. We have included some tasty combinations to add to your colorful palette of foods as you "eat for two."

## GREEN ● LIGHT

In addition to water, which is the best beverage, two of the next best beverages during pregnancy are green tea and cranberry juice. Green tea is terrific over ice or hot (add a touch of honey if you prefer) and carries great antioxidants. Cranberry juice (not the cocktail or juice drink variety) is perfect for good urinary tract health. Try diluting the juice with seltzer or water to reduce the high sugar content.

### Eggs and Spinach

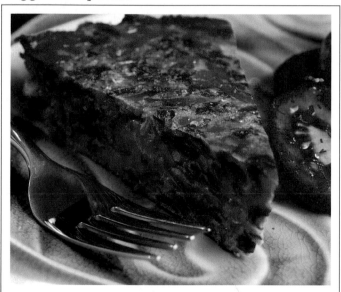

- This "eating for two" combo starts a great quiche for breakfast, lunch, or dinner.

- Eggs carry both protein and choline (in the yolk).

- A deficiency in choline can cause a deficiency in folic acid, which is a vital nutrient for pregnancy.

- Spinach is hands down one of the best food sources of vitamins K and A.

### Beef and Red Beans

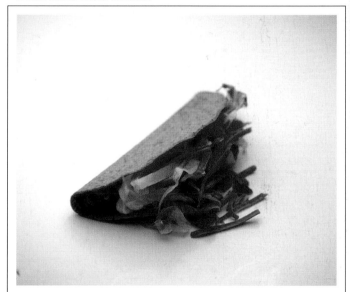

- This combo favorite is great in a taco or on a salad for lunch or dinner.

- The beef is chock-full of protein, vitamin B12, and iron.

- Red beans add fiber, protein, and folic acid to your diet.

- Choose chicken or turkey breast instead of beef if your cholesterol is high.

# IRON, CALCIUM, & PROTEIN

## You and your baby need iron, calcium, and protein for healthy tissues and bones

Three of the most critical nutrients for your pregnancy diet are iron, calcium, and protein. Your body needs iron for additional stores of blood. Iron is also needed to supply stores in the baby's liver. If you need to get more iron in your diet, some of your best food choices are meats such as beef and liver. Non-meat sources of iron include leafy green vegetables and cereals. You will need about thirty milligrams of iron each day during pregnancy.

Calcium is used to strengthen both your and your baby's skeletal system as well as teeth. Most women will need about 1,000 to 1,300 milligrams of calcium per day during pregnancy. While the best food sources of calcium come from

### Bran Flakes

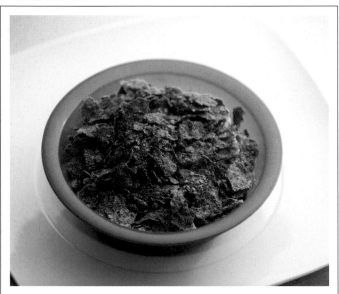

- Read labels on breakfast cereals for those that are high in iron.

- Some cereals, such as bran flakes, carry almost 50 percent of the daily iron you need in your pregnancy diet.

- Fortified cereals, such as bran flakes, are a good alternative to meat sources of iron.

- Bran cereals have the added benefit of folic acid and are also a good source of fiber.

### Skim Milk

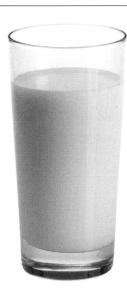

- Skim milk is one of the best sources of calcium for your pregnancy diet.

- It is definitely worth buying the organic brand of skim milk to avoid the hormones and antibiotics in milk.

- Skim milk is also a good source of protein.

- Don't forget that skim milk has the same nutritional value as whole milk, without any fat.

dairy, such as skim milk, yogurt and cheese, you can also get calcium from leafy green vegetables such as spinach, sardines, and salmon. Talk to your care provider to see whether you might need a calcium and/or vitamin D supplement.

Protein is a building block for pregnancy, as new cells are growing throughout the entire nine months. Protein is also a key player in the production of breast milk. The recommended amount of protein during pregnancy is about 60 grams each day. Some of the best sources of protein that you can include in your diet are lean beef, turkey, chicken, eggs, beans, and nuts.

⋯⋯⋯⋯⋯⋯ GREEN ● LIGHT ⋯⋯⋯⋯⋯⋯

One of the most common complaints during pregnancy is constipation. Mothers may find that getting approximately 40 grams of fiber a day can help relieve constipation symptoms. Fiber-rich foods include bran cereal, oatmeal, whole-grain breads, dried fruit such as prunes, beans, lentils, sweet potatoes, and all salad vegetables.

## Almonds

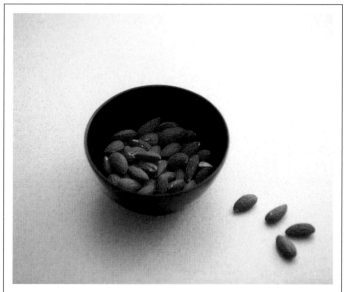

- Almonds are a good non-meat source of protein, with 20 grams for a ¼ cup serving.

- Almonds also contain good amounts of fiber, calcium, and vitamin E.

- Almonds are portable and easy to store in a zip top bag in your purse for quick snacking.

- The only downside of almonds is that they are very high in fat.

## Turkey

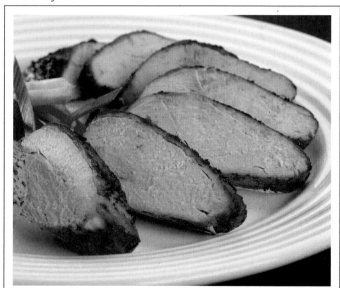

- The white meat in turkey is a great meat source of protein for your diet.

- Unlike beef, turkey is low in fat while giving you close to 30 grams of protein for each 3½-ounce serving.

- Turkey also has twice as much iron as chicken.

- Of all the meats, including pork, veal, beef, and chicken, turkey has the lowest amount of cholesterol per ounce.

15

# BENEFITS OF FOLIC ACID

## Folic acid is essential to your pregnancy diet in preventing spinal defects

Touted as one of the most crucial vitamins for a healthy pregnancy, folic acid has been proven to reduce the incidence of neural tube (spinal cord and some brain) defects in babies. For your baby's neural tube to close properly within the first month of pregnancy, you will need to have an adequate supply of folic acid onboard. In fact, experts now recommend that women start taking folic acid in the planning stages of pregnancy, at least two months before conception.

This water-soluble B vitamin can be found in foods such as fortified cereals and grains, green leafy vegetables, broccoli, asparagus, lentils, pinto beans, and papaya. Your goal should be to get about 1,000 micrograms of folic acid daily during

*Lentils*

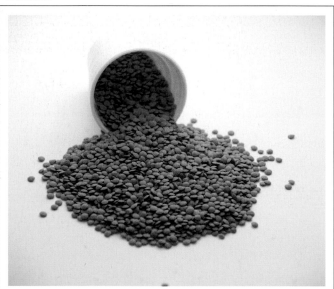

- Lentils are a member of the legume family and are easy to prepare in many recipes.

- They are jam-packed with folic acid and also add fiber to your diet.

- Lentils absorb flavors and spices, which is one reason why lentil soup is a favorite.

- If you are trying to cut back on your grocery bill, lentils are a steal at around $1 per one-pound bag.

*Asparagus*

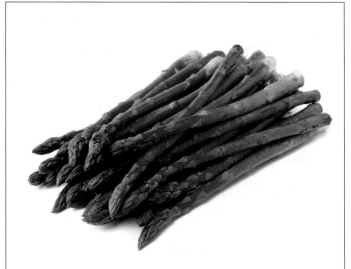

- This flavorful vegetable has more folic acid per serving than any other vegetable.

- One ½-cup serving of asparagus gives an expectant mother about one-third of her daily requirement of folic acid.

- Asparagus also has a great deal of vitamin K and some vitamin C to boot.

- This vegetable contains a special carbohydrate called inulin that helps to increase the good bacteria in our digestive system.

your pregnancy, and at least 400 micrograms daily before you conceive.

It's best to eat folic acid–rich vegetables raw since cooking reduces the amount of folic acid content. Eating foods that are high in vitamin C, will also help increase your body's ability to absorb folic acid.

## Enriched Bread

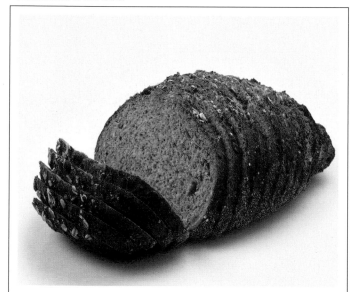

- Breads or flours are often enriched with folic acid to prevent birth defects.

- One slice of bread contains about 15 micrograms of folic acid.

- Look for breads that are also made from whole grains and contain at least 2 grams of fiber per slice. The best bread choices are those whose first ingredient is whole-wheat flour.

- One study has even shown that adding breads enriched with folic acid to your diet may help reduce depression.

## Enriched Cereal

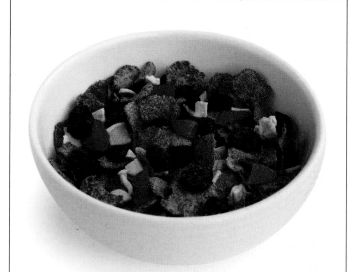

- The FDA requires that cereal, bread, and pasta be enriched with folic acid.

- A number of breakfast cereals contain close to a full day's supply of folic acid.

- Remember that expectant mothers need almost 200 micrograms more than the non-pregnant recommendation of folic acid (600 micrograms).

- Look for other healthy ingredients when making cereal choices such as iron, protein, and at least 5 grams of dietary fiber per serving.

# VITAMINS B6 & B12
## These two water-soluble vitamins help your body metabolize protein, fats, and carbs

Two of the most important water-soluble vitamins necessary for a healthy pregnancy are vitamins B6 and B12. Vitamin B6, known as pyridoxine, is used in a host of nervous system activities. It is needed in more than one hundred enzymatic reactions including your body's ability to metabolize protein. Since women of reproductive age are among the most at

risk for vitamin B6 deficiencies, be sure to talk with your care provider if you have any concerns about your own levels.

Low levels of vitamin B6 have also been associated with mothers who develop pregnancy-induced hypertension. The recommended daily amount of vitamin B6 is 1.9 milligrams daily during pregnancy. Foods rich in vitamin B6 that you

*Bananas*

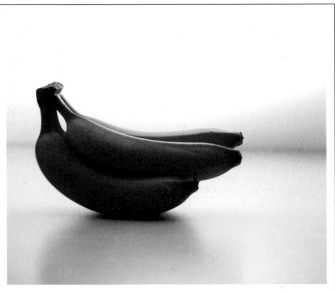

- Bananas are a convenient source of vitamin B6.

- They contain about 40 percent of your daily recommended amount of vitamin B6.

- You might be surprised to learn that bananas also contain about 6 grams of dietary fiber apiece.

- They also have a decent amount of vitamin C, potassium, and magnesium.

*Chicken*

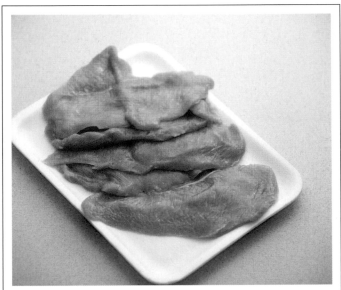

- One serving of chicken (half a chicken breast) contains about 25 percent of your recommended amount of vitamin B6.

- Chicken is a great source of protein, with a whopping 27 grams per serving.

- You can also get 60 grams of omega-3 fatty acids from one serving of chicken, which may help to reduce heart disease and lower high blood pressure.

- Be sure to trim off extra fat and stay away from fried chicken, to reduce excess calories from fat.

can easily add to your diet include yellowfin tuna, bananas, chicken, liver, and turkey. Smaller amounts of B6 are found in grains, nuts, seeds, and beans. Vitamin B12 helps your nerve cells to grow properly. Available from animal sources, this vitamin helps metabolize fats, proteins, and carbohydrates. The recommended amount of vitamin B12 in your pregnancy diet is 2.6 micrograms each day. By far the best food source of vitamin B12 is liver, although you can also get a good quantity from foods like salmon, snapper, venison, and beef as well as milk and milk byproducts.

## Salmon

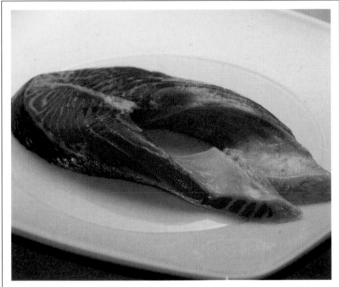

- Salmon is a great source of both vitamin B6 and vitamin B12.

- It has a good supply of additional minerals including selenium, phosphorus, and potassium.

- A single serving of salmon carries about 40 grams of protein and is "swimming" in omega-3.

- One downside is that salmon is loaded with fat, so be sure to vary your salmon intake with other low-fat protein choices.

## Safe Fishes for Pregnancy

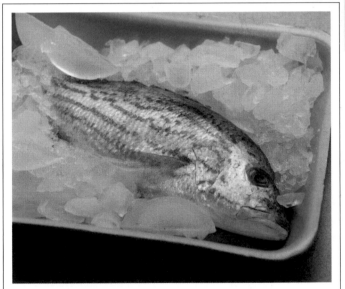

- Eating fish is one of the best ways to add healthy protein to your pregnancy diet.

- When selecting fish for your pregnancy diet, look for smaller fishes such as flounder, catfish, tilapia, and shellfish.

- Larger predator fishes such as swordfish, tilefish, King mackerel, and shark can contain unsafe amounts of mercury.

- The FDA recommends that pregnant women can safely eat about 6 ounces of canned tuna per week.

# VITAMINS A & C

## Vitamins A and C help you and your baby grow healthy cell tissue during your pregnancy

Noteworthy vitamins to add to your healthy pregnancy diet include both vitamins A and C. Vitamin A is a fat-soluble vitamin and is significant in developing healthy cell tissue. Eating the right amount of vitamin A helps you to grow strong bones, maintain healthy skin, and even aids with night vision. Some of the best sources of vitamin A include

sweet potatoes, chili peppers, and dark leafy vegetables such as Swiss chard and spinach. You should be getting approximately 1,000 RE (retimolequivalents) or 3,300 IU of vitamin A daily from supplements.

Also known as ascorbic acid, vitamin C is a water-soluble vitamin. During pregnancy it is a vitamin that is crucial in

### Sweet Potatoes

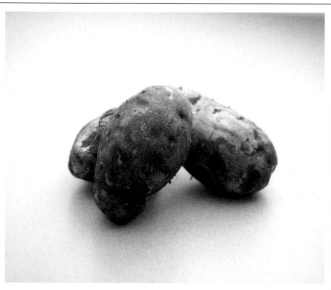

- If you want to add vitamin A to your diet, look no further. One cup of sweet potatoes has all of the vitamin A you need in just one serving.

- Sweet potatoes are also packed with vitamin B6 and vitamin C.

- They are also a good source of dietary fiber.

- Bake sweet potatoes by pricking potatoes a few times with a fork; place on baking sheet, bake at 400 degrees F for fifty to sixty minutes until soft.

### Swiss Chard

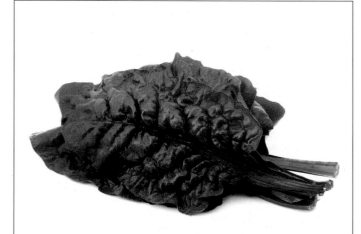

- Swiss chard is a lesser-known leafy vegetable that is similar to spinach but with more flavor.

- It is loaded with vitamin A and some vitamin C.

- Swiss chard even has a decent amount of fiber, potassium, and manganese.

- It can be cooked by boiling it, draining it well, chopping it, and adding a bit of salt for added flavor.

20

growing healthy and strong cell tissue. It also helps your body to form connective tissue. If you are concerned about getting enough iron, eating foods rich in vitamin C will help your body to absorb the iron in your diet. You will need about 70 milligrams of this multipurpose vitamin every day during pregnancy. Great sources of vitamin C include all fruits and vegetables. Eating one cup of sliced strawberries is about 81 milligrams, the equivalent of how much vitamin C you need every day.

*Broccoli*

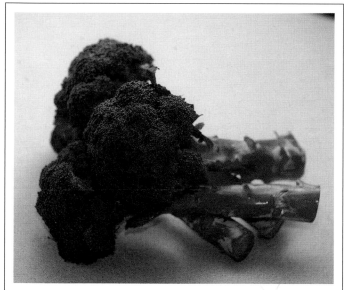

- Broccoli is often at the top of the list of healthiest foods.

- One serving has more than 100 percent of your total recommended amount of vitamin C.

- Broccoli also has good amounts of vitamin K, folic acid, and manganese.

- It can easily be added to salads, eaten raw with ranch dressing, or cooked to add with your dinner.

*Papaya*

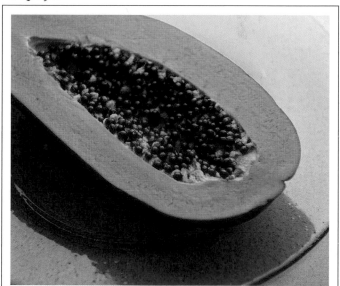

- One cup of papaya packs in 86 milligrams of vitamin C, which more than meets your daily needs for this vitamin.

- A single serving is about the equivalent of one small papaya.

- It also has the benefit of adding vitamin A and folic acid to your diet.

- Papayas contain papain, which aids digestion.

# CRAVINGS DURING PREGNANCY

## Having a food craving does not always mean your body is craving certain nutrients

If you are craving pickles and ice cream or french fries, you are not alone! It is not uncommon to crave desserts, food loaded with carbs, creamy foods, or foods high in sodium or fat. One problem with eating too much of these foods is that you fill your stomach with empty calories and do not get proper nutrients that you and your baby need. Many of these foods can also cause you to gain too much weight during pregnancy. Rather than making fries or ice cream sundaes a part of your daily diet, think of them as an occasional indulgence.

You might have heard that cravings encourage the mother to eat more of what her body may be lacking. While this may be true for a mother with a vegetarian diet who craves meat,

Healthier Substitutes for Cravings

• Low-fat frozen yogurt

• Hard cheese and whole-grain crackers

• Raw vegetables with low-fat dressing

• Tortilla chips with salsa

• Whole-wheat fig bars

• Air-popped popcorn

*Frozen Yogurt*

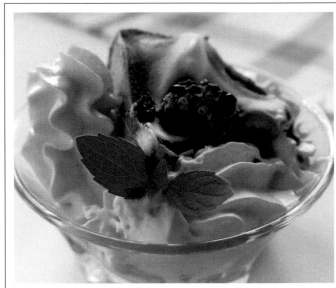

• For a lower-calorie dessert craving, nonfat frozen yogurt might be better than high-fat ice cream or milkshakes.

• Look for some of the nonfat varieties of frozen yogurt to get some of the benefit of calcium.

• You can usually get a little bit of protein as well from many frozen yogurt varieties.

• Add some fresh fruit to boost up your vitamins.

in other cases this theory does not hold up. This is definitely not true with mothers who crave junk food or non-food items (see sidebar).

Cravings may also play a role in our children's eating habits later. Recent studies support what anecdotal evidence has long suggested: the flavors of what you eat wind up in your amniotic fluid, so you are giving your baby a first taste of the vegetable or curry you are craving. Don't be surprised if later your child gravitates to those same foods you ate frequently during pregnancy.

·············· YELLOW ● LIGHT ··············

If you crave non-food substances like dirt, clay, and starch, this is known as pica. One possible reason for women to crave these unusual things could be a low supply of iron. You should give your care provider a call if you find that you are craving these non-food substances.

## Crackers and Cheese

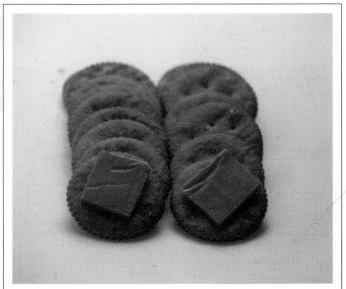

- Salty cravings can be satisfied with some healthy organic hard cheeses, such as cheddar, served with whole-grain crackers.

- Even though cheese is an excellent source of calcium and protein, it is loaded with fat, so eat it in moderation!

- Look for crackers that are made from whole grains and are high in fiber.

## Spice It Up

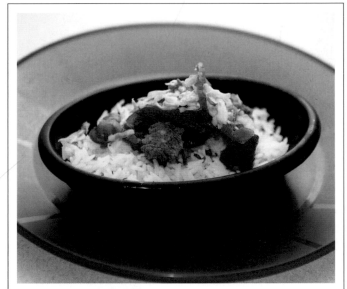

- If you crave foods with a kick and can tolerate them, there is no reason to stop eating them.

- In some cultures, these flavorful spices are a typical fixture in the diet and mothers eat them throughout pregnancy and breastfeeding.

- Spicy foods made from chilies contain capsaicin, and foods with curry contain curcumin.

- Both of these compounds contain anti-inflammatory and antioxidant components, so they are actually good for you.

# HEALTHY BREAKFAST TIPS

## Starting the day right at breakfast gives the pregnant mother fuel for her day

One reason that breakfast is considered to be the most important meal of the day is that you need the calories to get you started. Even on days when you are struggling to keep food down, keeping a small amount of food in your stomach all day does help. Some of our favorites for breakfast include a protein, a carbohydrate, and a fruit. Pancakes are a favorite because they digest easily and keep well in the freezer in a sealed container. You can also add fruit or berries while you are cooking the pancakes or just pile them on top. Add just a touch of real maple syrup rather than the artificial stuff. You can also add a bit more protein such a nitrate-free turkey bacon.

### Tips for Eating When You Just Can't

- Keep saltines at your bedside and eat a few before you get up.

- Sip fluids slowly throughout your day rather than taking large gulps.

- Always keep a small amount of food in your stomach.

- Bring small snacks when you are in a hurry.

*Blueberry Pancakes*

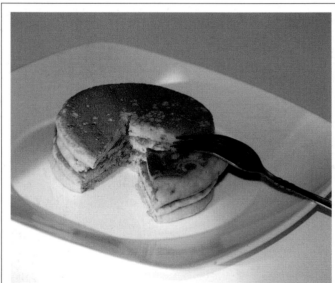

### Ingredients

Pancake mix
Egg(s)
Blueberries
Maple syrup
Butter if desired
Turkey bacon (no nitrates)

Cook bacon in a frying pan or in the microwave.

Mix pancake mix with water and eggs. Ladle batter onto a frying pan or electric griddle. Place blueberries on each pancake; flip when they bubble and are golden underneath. Add butter and maple syrup to taste. Serve with bacon and fruit.

Eggs are easy to fix and give you a good source of protein to give you energy to start your day. You can add a touch of sweet onion to your scrambled egg recipe for some flavor. Add fruit and some wheat toast and you are fueled up for the morning.

If you are wondering whether or not it is safe to add a cup of coffee to your breakfast menu, the answer might surprise you.

Prior recommendations were to avoid large quantities of caffeine and that a cup or two of coffee a day was safe.

However, new research has found that even caffeine levels of 100 milligrams per day, or the equivalent of one cup drip coffee increased the mother's risk of having a baby with a low birth weight. It is safest to reduce or eliminate your intake of caffeine throughout pregnancy.

## Scrambled Eggs

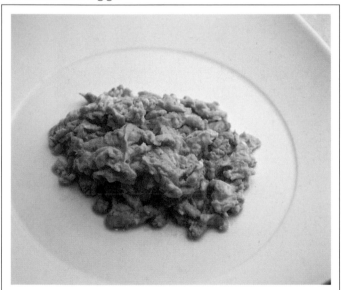

### Ingredients

2 eggs
Chopped onion
Whole-grain toast
Sliced fruit (cantaloupe, straw-berries, oranges, raspberries, papaya)

Sauté amount of chopped onion you desire until golden and soft. Add the eggs and scramble. Serve with toast (and butter if desired) and fruit.

## Yogurt Parfait

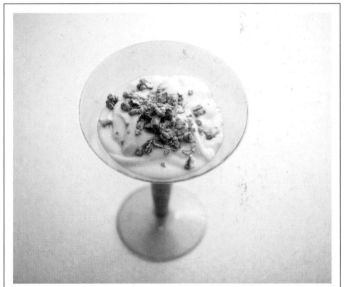

- A favorite breakfast for those mornings when you slept through your alarm is organic low-fat plain or vanilla yogurt.

- Mix the yogurt with any kind of berries or other fruit.

- Add a few tablespoons of granola. You could also substitute nuts instead of granola to add additional protein.

- This parfait makes a healthy breakfast when you don't have the time to cook any-thing. Enjoy!

# LUNCH ON THE GO
## Eating healthy at lunch is easy for moms-to-be with these great recipes

Lunch may be one of the most difficult meals for the expectant mother to pull together easily without being tempted to go for the drive-through option. Planning a little bit ahead for a healthy meal at lunchtime with a protein, vegetable or fruit, and carbohydrate is do-able even for the busy mother-to-be on the go. If you prefer a lighter meal such as a salad for lunch, be sure to add some meat, fish, or nuts for additional protein. You might find that warm foods such as soups or stews may even be more satisfying regardless of the season. If you have more time on the weekends, you can cook a large quantity of your favorite soup or stew and then freeze it in serving-size plastic containers to microwave and enjoy at

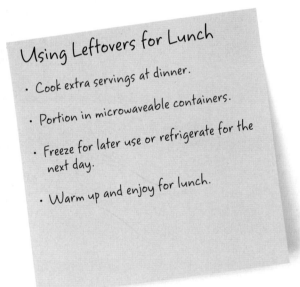

**Using Leftovers for Lunch**

- Cook extra servings at dinner.
- Portion in microwaveable containers.
- Freeze for later use or refrigerate for the next day.
- Warm up and enjoy for lunch.

*Southwestern Chicken Wrap*

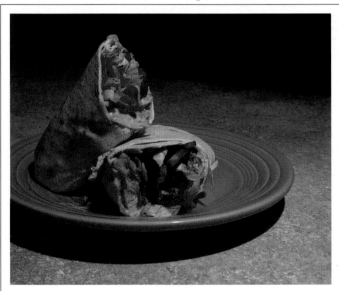

### Ingredients

1½ cups chopped cooked chicken
½ cup chunky salsa
1 15-ounce can black beans, rinsed and drained
1 7-ounce can whole-kernel corn, drained
6 fat-free flour tortillas
⅓ cup low-fat sour cream
½ cup shredded lettuce

Mix chicken, ½ cup salsa, beans, and corn in medium bowl; divide evenly among tortillas.

Spread chicken mixture to within 2 inches of bottom of each tortilla. Top with sour cream and lettuce.

lunchtime. Be wary of ready-made soups in microwavable containers available at your grocery store, since they can be very high in sodium. Sandwiches made on whole-grain breads that include a protein and paired up with a fruit or vegetable are quick to throw together before you head out to work. Another fun way to eat lunch on the go is to make a wrap.

For easy wrap-making, fold one end of the tortilla up about 1 inch over the filling; fold right and left sides over folded end, overlapping. Then fold the remaining end down. Some favorite wrap ingredients include meats, cheeses, shredded carrots or other raw vegetables, sliced tomatoes, chopped lettuce, and flavorings such as onions, hummus, and guacamole.

## Beef Vegetable Stew

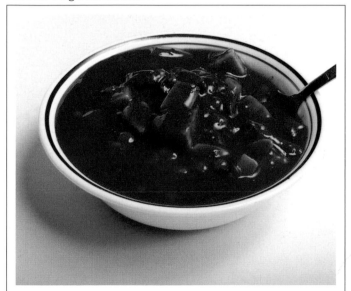

### Ingredients

1 pound cut up organic beef
3 tablespoons flour
1 tablespoon olive oil
28-ounce can diced tomatoes
1 large sweet onion, chopped
4 chopped cloves garlic
1 cup beef broth
4 cups sliced carrots
3 large potatoes, cut in pieces
1 cup cut green beans

1 tablespoon cornstarch
1 tablespoon water

Mix flour with beef, brown in oil. Mix remaining ingredients except water and cornstarch in slow cooker.

Add beef; cover. Cook on high 4 to 6 hours. Mix cornstarch with water; add to stew.

## Healthy Sandwich

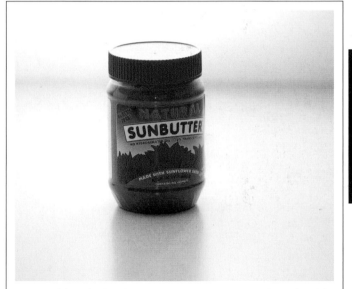

- A quick lunch idea that is packed with nutrients is a healthier twist on a peanut butter and jelly sandwich.

- Start with sunflower seed butter, add organic strawberry or blueberry preserves on whole-grain bread and include carrot sticks on the side.

- Expectant mothers should be limiting their intake of peanut butter, so we suggest sunflower seed butter as a healthy substitute.

- It's packed with magnesium for strong bones and vitamin E, a powerful antioxidant.

# NUTRITIOUS & DELICIOUS DINNERS

## Using your slow cooker during pregnancy is one way to make dinner almost effortless

Does your schedule allow you neither the time nor the energy to spend hours in the kitchen cooking over a hot stove? Do you get home from work and just want to curl up on the couch and have someone else make your dinner? Add to your fatigue the task of trying to make a healthy dinner in just minutes, and the task seems nearly impossible.

This doesn't leave you with many meal choices that are both quick and healthy for your body and your growing baby.

An easy solution for quick and nutritious dinners during pregnancy is using your slow cooker. If you do not own one, they are well worth the $50 price tag. Many times all you need to do is throw in a few vegetables, meat, and spices and

### Slow Cooker Tips

- Recipe cooking times vary, so monitor your meals the first few times you use the slow cooker.

- Place root vegetables on the bottom.

- Cook on high for one hour, then turn to low for food safety.

- Defrost all frozen foods before placing in slow cooker.

- Add spices generously since the flavors get watered down.

- Fill cooker only one-half to two-thirds full.

- Save the juices and vegetables for soup base.

### Slow Cooker

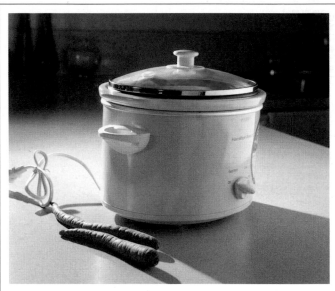

- Slow cookers are one of the best ways to save on your grocery bill as well as hours in the kitchen.

- Find one with a removable pot on the inside.

- You can purchase slow cookers in the kitchen section of nearly any department store.

- Prices vary anywhere from $40 for a smaller 5-quart slow cooker to over $100 for a 7-quart stainless-steel model.

some broth and you have dinner waiting for you when you walk in the door. There are tons of slow cooker recipes online and in recipe books to choose from. After you get more comfortable in preparing meals with your slow cooker, you may begin to create your own recipes.

## Chicken Dinner in a Pot

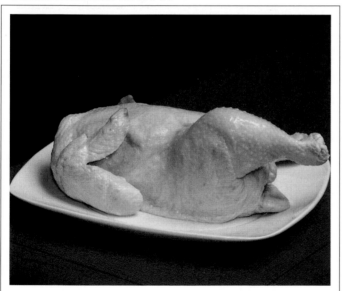

### Ingredients

1 3–5-pound whole (broiler, fryer) organic chicken
1–2 cups chicken broth
2–3 carrots, sliced
1 medium sweet onion, chopped
2 stalks celery with leaves, chopped
3 teaspoons salt
Pepper

2 cloves garlic, pressed
2 teaspoons parsley

Place broth, vegetables in bottom of slow cooker. Rinse chicken; remove organ meats. Place chicken on top of vegetables, add spices, salt, and pepper. Cover; cook on high 4 to 5 hours or low 7 to 8 hours.

## Beef Brisket

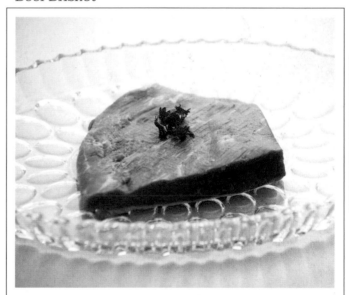

### Ingredients

3–5-pound brisket
1 large sweet onion
Bottled or homemade barbecue sauce (enough to cover the meat)
3–4 potatoes, cooked and mashed
Green beans or other green vegetable

Cut brisket in half to fit slow cooker if needed. Add onion and barbecue sauce. Cover and cook on low for about 8 to 10 hours. During the last 30 minutes of cooking the meat, peel, boil, and mash potatoes and cook green vegetable. Use juices to make gravy.

# QUICK & HEALTHY SNACKS

## Snacks can be a healthy alternative when eating a full meal is not practical

Eating healthy snacks often becomes a necessity in both the first and last trimesters of your pregnancy. Morning sickness can make it tough to keep a big meal down in your first trimester, so eating smaller amounts throughout your day sometimes helps. As the baby takes up more and more space, your stomach can hold only smaller amounts of food

in your last trimester. Grazing on healthy snacks during the day seems to be a popular solution for many of the digestive upsets that go along with being pregnant, no matter where you are in your pregnancy.

Some of the best snacks are those that you can take along with you and do not require refrigeration. Favorite snacks

### Fruit and Nut Mix

- I cup almonds

- I cup unsalted dry-roasted peanuts

- I cup raisins or dried fruit (your choice)

- I cup dark chocolate chips

- Mix and enjoy.

- Makes 8 servings

### Dried Fruit

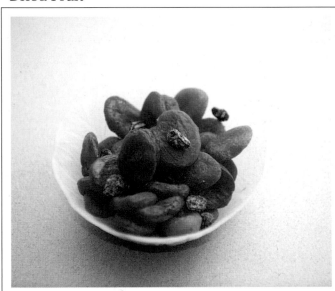

- Even though dried fruit can be more convenient to take along, it's higher in calories and sometimes has less nutritional value than its fresh-fruit counterparts.

- Look for dried fruit with natural sweeteners such as apple juice rather than refined sugar or corn syrup.

- Dried fruit adds fiber and iron to your diet so it makes for a healthy snack to take on the go.

- It is also a good source of potassium, magnesium, and many vitamins including A and B1, 2, and 3.

include dried fruits, granola/trail mix, nuts (almonds are one of the healthiest!), whole-grain crackers, breakfast cereal, and pretzels.

Fresh fruit such as an orange, apple, or banana is also a quick and nutritious snack to grab on your way out the door if you need to add more fruit to your diet that day. If you need a protein snack, you can boil several eggs at a time so that you can just grab one out of the refrigerator as you head out. Some mothers enjoy granola or energy bars, but be sure to read the labels since some protein bars may contain ingredients that are less than healthy, such as high-fructose corn syrup or tons of unnecessary sugar. If you have a small cooler bag, you can add some hard cheese or yogurt to your healthy snack list.

## Hard-Boiled Eggs

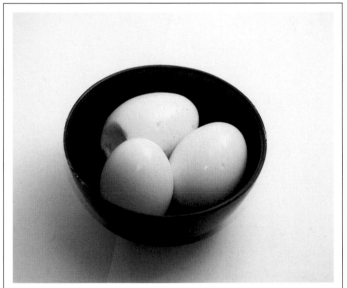

- It can be easy to undercook or overcook hard-boiled eggs.

- For perfect hard-boiled eggs, place eggs in a pot with water completely covering the eggs.

- Heat pot to boiling and boil for ten minutes. Immediately cool eggs with cold running water.

- Refrigerate and enjoy for a perfect snack!

## Snacks

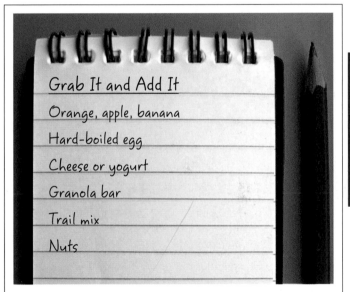

Grab It and Add It
Orange, apple, banana
Hard-boiled egg
Cheese or yogurt
Granola bar
Trail mix
Nuts

- Snacks can be an area where pregnant moms need to be cautious of adding empty calories.

- Rather than grabbing french fries or potato chips, think ahead to healthy snacks you can take with you.

- Munching on some trail mix or a piece of fruit will help if you have to wait longer between meals.

- Not to mention, healthy snacking helps to curb early pregnancy morning sickness.

# MOMS WITH SPECIAL DIETS

## Lactose-intolerant or vegan moms may be lacking calcium and other nutrients in their diets

Making sure you are getting all of the proper nutrients and vitamins during pregnancy can be more challenging for mothers with special diets. One of the most common dietary problems is lactose intolerance. Pregnant women who cannot digest dairy may have difficulty getting the total amount of calcium that they need every day. While other food sources

such as broccoli and spinach contain calcium, these vegetable sources don't have as much calcium per serving. Be sure to contact your care provider if you are lactose intolerant as you may need to take a calcium supplement.

If you have a strict vegan diet and do not consume any food from animal sources, you will need to be more aware of your

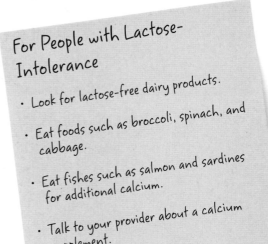

For People with Lactose-Intolerance

- Look for lactose-free dairy products.

- Eat foods such as broccoli, spinach, and cabbage.

- Eat fishes such as salmon and sardines for additional calcium.

- Talk to your provider about a calcium supplement.

*Fruits and Vegetables*

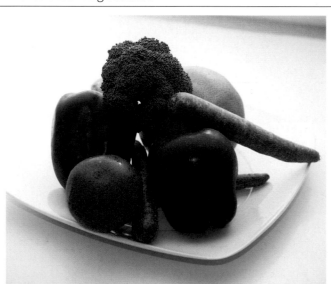

- Moms with lactose intolerance should add foods rich in calcium to their diets.

- Non-dairy food sources that are high in calcium include cabbage and bok choy.

- Other foods rich in calcium include turnip greens, broc-coli, collard greens, kale, Swiss chard, celery, and oranges.

- Eat your calcium-rich foods throughout your day rather than all at once since your body best manages about 500 milligrams of calcium at a time.

intake of calcium, vitamin B12, iron, and protein. You can add calcium to your diet by eating dark leafy vegetables, sesame butter, sea vegetables, and grains such as tapioca. In order to get non-meat sources of vitamin B12, you can drink enriched soy milk or talk to your caregiver about a supplement. Iron sources can be found in enriched breads, dark green vegetables, legumes, and dried fruit. Plant sources of protein for a vegetarian diet include grains, nuts, legumes, and seeds.

Soy is a common ingredient in breads, snack bars, vegetarian foods, and cereals. These products are often labeled "high protein." Soy is also a popular ingredient in infant formula. However, soy contains isoflavone, an estrogen-like compound that is associated with thyroid disease and infertility for both men and women. Given that long-term studies on the effects of soy are limited, it makes sense to reduce the amount of soy in your family's diet.

## Vegan Diet

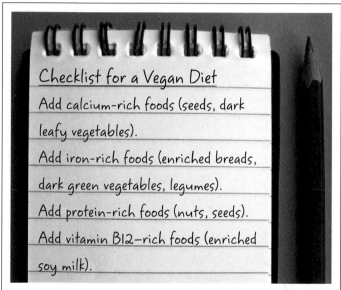

Checklist for a Vegan Diet

Add calcium-rich foods (seeds, dark leafy vegetables).

Add iron-rich foods (enriched breads, dark green vegetables, legumes).

Add protein-rich foods (nuts, seeds).

Add vitamin B12-rich foods (enriched soy milk).

- Vegan Diet: consists of only plant-based foods with no meat or dairy.

- Lacto-Vegetarian Diet: consists of plant-based foods plus dairy such as cheese and milk. It excludes meats.

- Ovo-Vegetarian Diet: allows eggs in addition to plant-based foods, but does not include meat, dairy, or fish.

- Lacto-Ovo Vegetarian Diet: includes eating eggs and dairy with plant-based foods but does not allow meat or fish.

## Grains, Beans, and Nuts

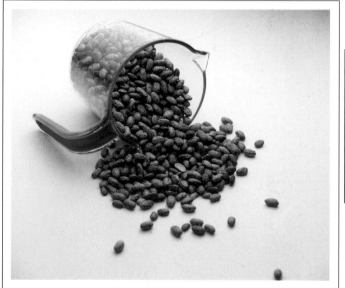

- For expectant mothers who have vegetarian diets, be sure you are adding non-meat sources of protein such as enriched breads and pasta, legumes, and nuts.

- Some whole-grain breads can have as much as 10 grams of protein per slice.

- Legumes are also great sources of protein and include lentils, beans, and peas.

- One serving of pinto beans combined with a slice of enriched bread carries as much protein as one serving of red meat without the calories and saturated fat.

# READING LABELS
## Eating foods that are highly processed is not good for either mom or baby

The next time you are shopping for groceries, take a look around the store. The outside perimeter of the store typically has dairy, meats, breads, and produce. The inner aisles of the store contain shelf after shelf of pre-made, ready-to-eat, and highly processed foods. Some of these foods might have some nutrition, but one of the problems is that many contain long lists of ingredients that are hard to pronounce. Most of those multisyllabic ingredients are additives to enhance the flavor or the food, colorings to make the food more appealing to the eye, or preservatives to help the food last longer on the shelves. So there is actually a two-fold problem with highly processed foods: One is their lack of

**Grocery Store Dos and Don'ts**

- Avoid the middle section of the store.

- Avoid products with a long list of ingredients.

- Avoid products with preservatives.

- Avoid products that enhance flavor.

- Avoid products with dyes or coloring.

### Less Is More

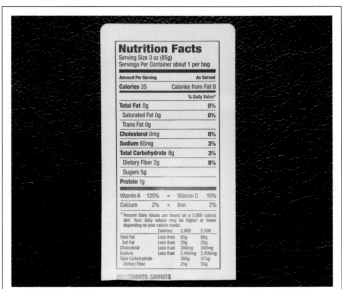

- If you read a label and you only see a few ingredients listed, the food has minimal processing and likely has few additives or preservatives.

- For example, organic butter comes from organic whole-milk cream and salt.

- Yet, some manufacturers tell us that substitutes for butter are healthier for us because they are lower in fat.

- The truth is that in moderation, butter may be the healthier food choice.

nutrition and the other is the potential harm from additives and preservatives.

The reality is that our diet today contains more and more chemicals and artificial ingredients and we are getting less and less nutrition. Some refer to this type of highly-processed food as "dead." While we do not have testing on all of the food additives in the grocery store in order to know their effects on baby, you and your baby will benefit by limiting your intake of processed foods. Since you may not have the option to make all of your foods from scratch, you should be a label reader.

•••••••••• YELLOW ● LIGHT ••••••••••

You might want to start reading labels in your bathroom as well. Cosmetics, skin-care products, toothpaste, shampoo, and deodorants also contain preservatives and chemicals. Believe it or not, even your prenatal vitamins may contain preservatives, so look for a brand that is free from additives and preservatives.

## Name That Ingredient

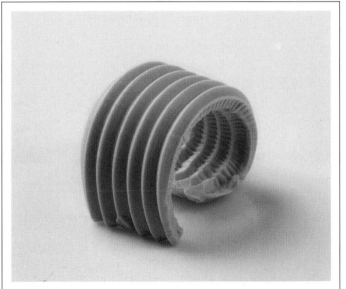

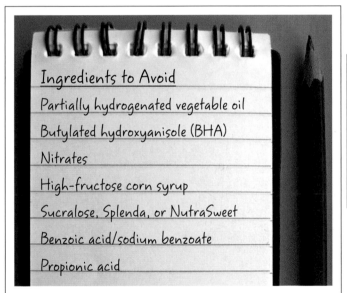

- Margarine has a host of ingredients, including mono- and diglycerides (emulsifiers to hold the ingredients together) and preservatives (sodium benzoate) to prevent the margarine from spoiling too soon.

- You may also see that butter flavors and artificial colors are added.

- We do not know the long-term health consequences of filling our bodies with all of these artificial chemicals.

- Expectant mothers should try to reduce their babies' exposure to these chemicals when possible.

**Ingredients to Avoid**
Partially hydrogenated vegetable oil
Butylated hydroxyanisole (BHA)
Nitrates
High-fructose corn syrup
Sucralose, Splenda, or NutraSweet
Benzoic acid/sodium benzoate
Propionic acid

- A good rule of thumb is to try to avoid products that contain these and other additives.

- Some of the biggest offenders that contain multiple chemicals are diet sodas and deli meats.

- Questions remain about the safety of artificial sweeteners during pregnancy.

- For that reason, it is best to limit or restrict your intake of artificial sweeteners while pregnant.

# EXERCISE GUIDELINES

## Making sure your exercise plan is safe before you start is important for today's expectant mothers

Staying active during pregnancy has many benefits, including relieving discomfort and staying toned for childbirth. If you are planning to continue your current exercise regimen or begin a new one, be sure to check with your care provider to see if your plan might need to be altered. As you continue into the latter months of pregnancy, if you begin to have any

preterm labor symptoms, your plan for exercise will need to be changed.

After you get the go-ahead from your physician or midwife, you might want to consider starting your exercise plan with walking, swimming, or other forms of low-impact aerobics during pregnancy. Ideally you should start slowly, with even

### Exercise Tips

- Check with your care provider first.
- Change your exercise plan if you have any preterm labor symptoms.
- Start with low-impact exercise such as walking.
- Exercise for ten minutes if just beginning.
- Continue to exercise three or more times each week.
- Reduce activity in last trimester if needed.

*Pregnancy Exercises*

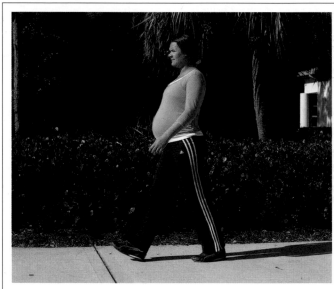

- Some of the best pregnancy exercise programs include walking, swimming, yoga, water aerobics, dancing, and stationary bicycling.

- These exercises are all low-impact and gentle enough to engage in throughout pregnancy.

- On occasion, your exercise program may need to change if complications occur.

- Remember to check in with your care provider should you have concerns about your level of exercise during pregnancy.

as little as ten minutes of exercise at a time, especially if this is a new form of exercise to you. Continue your exercise activity at least three times per week.

Be sure to wear comfortable and supportive clothing as you exercise, including shoes appropriate to your activity. Your shoe size often changes during pregnancy, so make sure you are fitted properly. By six to seven months of pregnancy, you may need to reduce your activity level as your center of gravity shifts and you become more unwieldy.

## Fitting Shoes

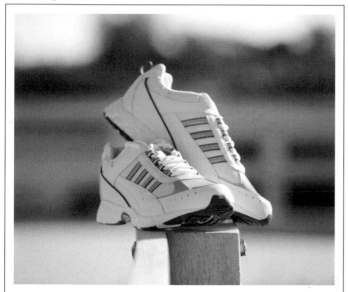

- Buy shoes at an athletic store so that you can be fitted properly.

- Wear the same type of sock you will wear during your pregnancy exercise. Have someone else measure your feet.

- Be sure you have at least half an inch of space between your biggest toe and the end of your shoe.

- Look for plenty of width space, and if you have wide feet, consider a men's size.

## Strength Training

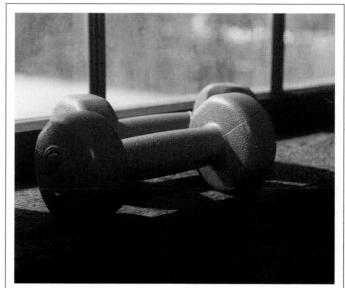

- Strength training during pregnancy is safe with some precautions.

- Do not lift weights while on your back. You may want to use a machine rather than free weights to avoid dropping weights.

- As your pregnancy progresses, you may need to lighten your weights.

- For extra help, look for classes offered at your local gym for weight lifting during pregnancy.

EXERCISE

# UNSAFE EXERCISES

## Mothers should not bounce or hold their breath while doing pregnancy exercises

You may have heard that you should avoid any exercise while lying on your back after your first trimester. The reason is that the weight of your uterus presses on the large blood vessels in your lower back, known as the vena cava and aorta. If the vena cava becomes constricted, it can slow the blood return from the lower part of your body to your heart, causing you to feel dizzy and short of breath and reduce blood flow to the uterus. Instead, you can prop yourself in a semi-upright position or lie on your side during exercise or sleep.

Activities and sports that are not considered to be safe during pregnancy include basketball, scuba-diving, water- or downhill skiing, gymnastics, horseback riding, soccer, and

Unsafe Exercises

- Lying on your back after the first trimester
- Horseback riding
- Downhill skiing
- Scuba diving
- Gymnastics
- High-impact sports

*Low-impact Exercise*

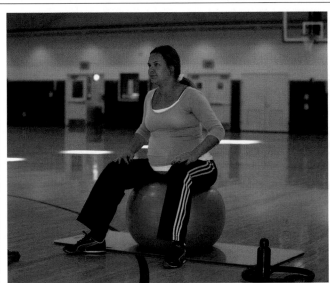

- Low-impact exercises such as walking and water aerobics are not jarring to your body and are less likely to result in injury.

- One study actually showed that mothers who participated in an aquarobics program used less pain medication during labor.

- If you have access to a gym, talk to a fitness trainer about gentle exercises that you can do during pregnancy to tone your body as well as improve cardiovascular health.

- The birth ball is a great tool for pregnancy exercise so be sure to take advantage of it.

other high-impact sports. It is also wise for expectant mothers to avoid strenuous exercise in high heat or humidity since raising your body temperature might be unsafe to your baby. Be careful not to bounce or hold your breath with your exercise or stretching activity.

The current recommendations by the American College of Obstetricians and Gynecologists (ACOG) state that if you can talk normally while you are exercising, your heart rate is at an acceptable level and need not be measured.

## Group Exercise

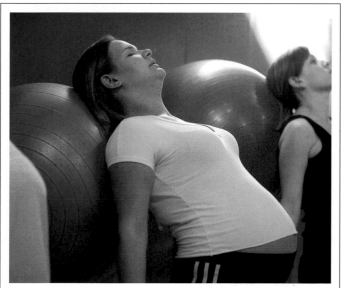

- You might find that scheduling your pregnancy exercise program at a certain time with a group of people helps you stay consistent.

- Exercise classes are also a great way to get extra help with pregnancy exercise.

- Or you might consider scheduling a walk in the morning or late afternoon with a friend.

- Group exercise is one way to hold you accountable for being consistent with your exercise during pregnancy.

When to Call Your Care Provider

- Vaginal bleeding

- Lightheadedness or dizziness

- Headache

- Increased shortness of breath

- Chest pain

- Muscle weakness

- Calf pain

- Uterine contractions

- Decreased movement of the baby

- Leaking vaginal fluid

EXERCISE

# PRE- & POST-EXERCISE TIPS

## Eating a light snack an hour after exercise is helpful for replenishing some lost energy

Warming up is essential for safe exercise to prevent expectant mothers from inadvertent injury. Before you begin exercising, be sure you are well hydrated. You might start with eight ounces of water and continue hydrating throughout your activity. About every twenty to thirty minutes of exercise, you should drink another eight ounces of water. Dress in layers so that you can peel off the outer layers as you warm up.

Some helpful warm-up exercises include doing head rolls from side-to-side (to relax your neck and shoulders); lunging with one foot about 2 feet in front of the other, stretch each arm above your head, separately and then both together; and the angry cat or pelvic tilt exercise, to stretch your lower

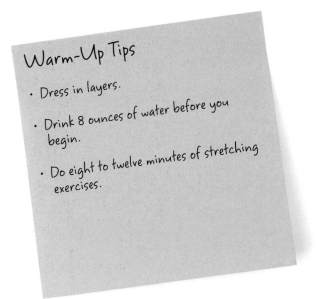

### Warm-Up Tips

- Dress in layers.
- Drink 8 ounces of water before you begin.
- Do eight to twelve minutes of stretching exercises.

*Post-exercise Fuel*

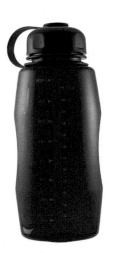

- Plenty of water and a nutritional snack are two of the best ways to replenish lost energy after exercise.

- Be sure to look for water bottles that are bisphenol A (BPA)-free.

- The jury is out about whether cold water is preferred over room temperature, but everyone agrees that drinking water is essential.

- You might enjoy a quick snack after exercise from our "Grab it and go" list in chapter three.

back muscles. You can do a pelvic tilt in a hands and knees position and rotate your pelvis up and forward until your back arches. Your warm-up should be about eight to twelve minutes in length.

Cooling down from your exercise is just as important as the warm-up. It helps your heart rate return slowly to normal, avoids dizziness when exercise stops too suddenly, and helps your muscles get rid of lactic acid buildup. After your activity, be sure to drink at least one more 8-ounce cup of water. Continue to walk and stretch slowly for at least five minutes, more if possible, after you finish exercising since it can take that long for your heart rate to return to normal. Depending on how strenuous your exercise is, you may need to continue to drink fluids for several hours to stay well hydrated. Be sure to add an extra layer of clothing or change into dry clothing if you are leaving the gym and heading into colder temperatures outside. Grabbing a light snack about an hour after you exercise can help your body recover from your workout. Wait until you have completely cooled down before heading into the shower to give your body a chance to get rid of the extra heat.

## Swimming

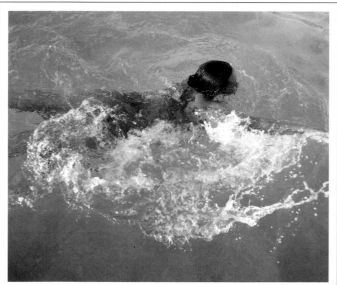

- Swimming at your community pool or gym is safe, but resist the urge to use the hot tub.

- Most hot tub temperatures will be higher than your body temperature and therefore will increase your own body temperature after a few minutes.

- When mother's body temperature increases, it can raise the baby's heart rate.

- The rise in the baby's heart rate increases stress on the baby's cardiovascular system.

### Cool-Down Tips

- Drink at least 8 ounces of water.
- Stretch for fifteen minutes.
- Add a layer of clothing.
- Eat a light snack.
- Cool down before showering.

EXERCISE

41

# BODY CHANGES DURING PREGNANCY

## The relaxin hormone helps to increase mother's flexibility during pregnancy and childbirth

While mothers know that their body changes in multiple ways during pregnancy and that they can injure themselves doing new activities, they may not know exactly how or why this happens.

The reason behind your loose joints and ligaments is an incredible hormone called relaxin. Relaxin is actually a member of the insulin family and is secreted by both males and females. In men it helps fertility by increasing the motility of the sperm in semen. During pregnancy relaxin peaks about 14 days after you conceive and then once again by the time you reach your due date. Researchers believe that it aids in the growth of your uterus and placenta and helps the little

### The Job of Relaxin

- Aids in implantation of pregnancy
- Helps uterus and placenta grow
- Widens pelvic joints and ligaments
- Softens cervix
- Relaxes uterus

### Pelvis Up Close

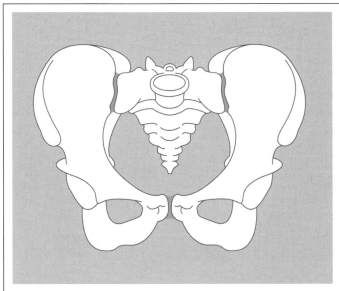

- The female pelvis is held together by a number of joints, including the pubic symphysis (pubic bone), the sacrococcygeal joint (attaching tail bone to the sacrum), and the sacroiliac joints, which attach the pelvis to the lower backbone.

- These joints and ligaments stretch and loosen due to relaxin during pregnancy.

- This loosening helps to make more room for your baby during pregnancy.

- As pelvic joints and ligaments stretch, it can be painful and discomforting.

embryo implant into your uterus. During labor, relaxin helps your baby pass through your pelvis more easily. It helps to widen your pubic ligament (making more space in the pelvis), soften your cervix, and relax your uterus. Relaxin may also play a role in the timing of when your water breaks when you are close to your due date. Studies have shown that artificial relaxin helped to prepare mothers' bodies for labor.

Since relaxin is present during pregnancy at ten times the normal amount, the over-stretching of your joints, muscles, and ligaments can be a cause of pain and discomfort for many expectant moms. Some mothers experience hip pain and lower back pain as a result of the increase in relaxin secreted during pregnancy. Also, your looser, more flexible body parts can make injury more likely to occur if you are not aware that you are stretching more than what is ideal. All the more reason you should avoid exercise your body is not used to as well as heavy lifting or straining in your activities around the house or at work. If you suspect you have pulled a muscle or sprained a ligament, contact your care provider for guidance.

## Looser Ligaments

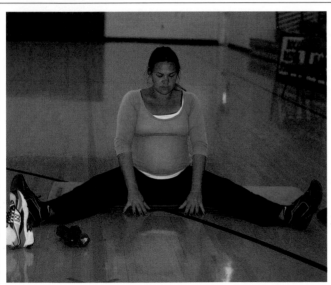

- During pregnancy, mothers may notice during exercise that their body feels looser and more flexible.

- However, relaxin can make it a bit more challenging to recognize right away when you might have "over-done" your exercise.

- Be sure that you go easy with any new form of exercise, until your body has had time to get used to it.

- Remember that relaxin will also increase again at the end of pregnancy to prepare your body for labor.

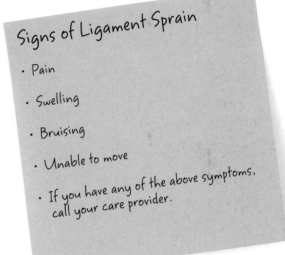

Signs of Ligament Sprain

- Pain

- Swelling

- Bruising

- Unable to move

- If you have any of the above symptoms, call your care provider.

# MANAGING DISCOMFORT

## Using a birthing ball instead of an office chair can strengthen your lower-back muscles

Is your back pain getting the best of you in your pregnancy? The sheer weight of the baby can cause your center of gravity to be shifted in such a way that you force your hips slightly forward, lean your shoulders back, and end up with the walk that looks like a "pregnancy waddle." Stretching your lower back with pelvic tilts, either standing or on all fours,

can strengthen these muscles and reduce your discomfort. Using a birthing ball instead of an office chair can also help you strengthen the muscles in your lower back.

Swelling is also common during pregnancy, especially in your ankles. You might notice swelling is worse in the warm weather months. Doing ankle rotations, one at a time, can

### Benefits of Toning Exercise

- Reduces back pain
- Reduces hip or pelvic discomfort
- Helps prevent injury
- Strengthens muscles
- Reduces swelling
- Increases circulation

### Birth Balls

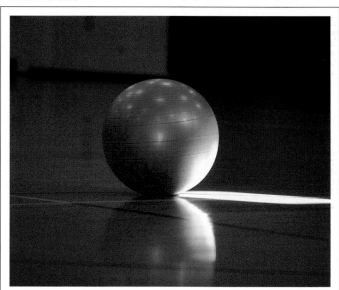

- Straddling a birth ball relaxes your pelvic floor and uses your back muscles more than a chair does.

- Lean over and "hug" the ball to stretch your lower back and ease back pain.

- They are sold as fitness or Pilates balls in sporting-goods or department stores.

- Cost is about $15 to $25.

help to increase circulation and reduce swelling. If you are noticing a sudden increase in swelling, especially in your face, hands, or feet, be sure to contact your care provider.

As your baby grows and takes up more space, your bladder can become irritated. It is common to have some leakage when you cough or sneeze. Pregnancy is an ideal time to start to strengthen your pelvic floor muscles by doing Kegel exercises. These are exercises in which you tighten and hold the muscles of your pelvic floor, just as you would if you were trying to stop from urinating.

•••••••••• YELLOW●LIGHT ••••••••••

If you are on bed rest for symptoms of preterm labor, even your bathroom privileges might be restricted, much less any other type of exercise! Check in with your care provider to see what stretching exercises can be done. Yoga might be used as a way to reduce stress and discomfort associated with being confined to bed rest. Gentle stretching is a good way to not only promote relaxation, but maintain strength and muscle tone.

## Toning and Stretching

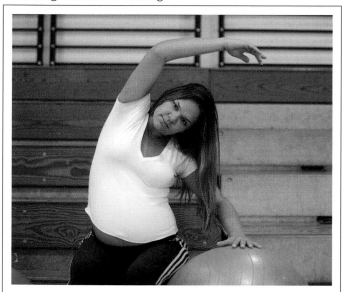

- Any pregnancy exercise that works on muscle groups brings more circulation to that area.

- If you do a lot of sitting at your job, be sure to get up every hour to stretch and move around to prevent your muscles from tightening up.

- Many women tend to hold tension in their upper back, shoulders, and neck area.

- Watch for places in your body where you hold tension, and stretch those areas often.

## Pelvic Floor

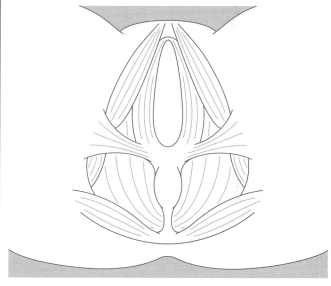

- The muscles of your pelvic floor support the weight of your baby and abdomen.

- These muscles can be weakened due to the additional weight of pregnancy.

- Pelvic floor exercises (called Kegels) should be practiced several times per day.

- Regular conditioning of these muscle groups can reduce bladder leakage.

EXERCISE

# EXERCISE MYTHS

## Mothers need to know fact from fiction when it comes to pregnancy exercise

Some folks believe that doing regular exercise during pregnancy will shorten your labor. Or maybe all it took was one athlete to have a phenomenally easy labor and then everyone wanted to cash in on their free ride. The reality is that, for some women, prenatal exercise could reduce the length of their labor. However, be careful to think of exercise as a formula that guarantees a short labor. Exercise can help increase your stamina during the long hours of early labor. Many mothers who are avid runners compare labor to their longest marathon! You may also find that staying active during pregnancy helps you bounce back more easily after birth.

Another myth is that exercising will take nutrients from your

**Benefits of Exercise**

- Reduces pregnancy discomforts
- Reduces risk of preterm labor
- Helps increase stamina for labor
- Helps in recovery from birth
- Healthy for baby

*Endorphins*

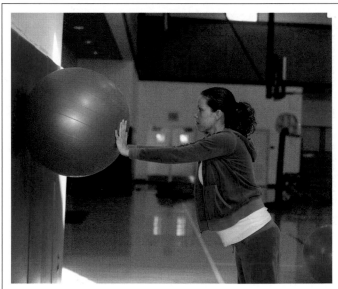

- When you exercise, your body releases endorphins that give you a wonderful sensation, also known as "runner's high."

- They are similar to opiates in that they also work as natural pain relievers.

- These endorphins help give you an energy boost to give you endurance, whether it is during exercise or labor.

- Other ways that endorphins are stimulated is through lovemaking, excitement, and even through acupuncture.

baby. While you do need to replenish your body with good hydration and healthy foods after you exercise, the most important way to make sure your baby has sufficient nutrients is to have a healthy diet and take prenatal vitamins.

Abdominal exercises should be safe to do as long as you do not have diastasis recti. Be careful not to do any abdominal exercises while lying on your back. Exercise your tummy muscles by doing a pelvic tilt in a standing position by leaning against a wall with your feet about shoulder-width apart, heels 12 inches from the wall, and your knees bent.

Another interesting benefit to exercise is that staying active may reduce your chances of having a preterm birth. Over 80,000 mothers participated in a study done in Copenhagen. One-third of the mothers stayed active during pregnancy with low-impact exercise such as walking, swimming, and hiking. Active mothers had a lower risk of having a preterm birth than those who were not.

## Exercise and Labor

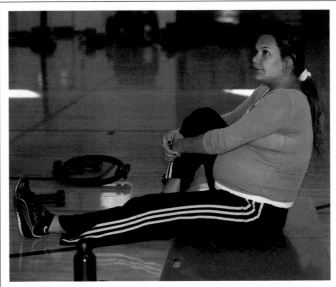

- Just like strenuous exercise, labor feels very much like you need to push yourself past the point where you think you can't go on.

- Working through each contraction takes a tremendous amount of physical energy.

- Childbirth also takes preparation, both physically and mentally for the task ahead.

- Perhaps that is one reason why many female athletes find that labor feels very much like the most intense workout of all.

## Checking for Diastasis Recti

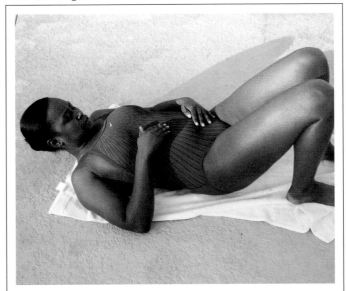

- Lie on the floor with your knees bent and feet on the floor. Put one hand behind your head.

- Place the other on your abdomen with your fingertips across your midline right at the level of your navel.

- Press your fingertips into your abdomen. Roll your upper body into a "crunch."

- Feel for both sides of this diastasis muscle on the right and left. Separation of more than two finger-widths is diastasis recti.

EXERCISE

# PREGNANCY GENETICS & VARIATIONS

## Chromosomes from each mother and father are responsible for the physical traits and health of each baby

Pregnancy is not just about physical changes in your body. It also involves incredibly complicated biological processes that are taking place even when you are unaware of them. Each of you brings twenty-three single chromosomes to your baby; twenty-three from the egg and twenty-three from the sperm cell. The egg contains twenty-two chromosomes plus one X chromosome. The sperm contains twenty-two chromosomes plus either an X or a Y chromosome, which will determine the gender of your baby. Once the ovum is fertilized by the sperm, it will contain forty-six chromosomes. These chromosomes play a role in the genetic makeup of your baby including gender, hair color, eye color, height, and other physical traits.

### Gender of Baby

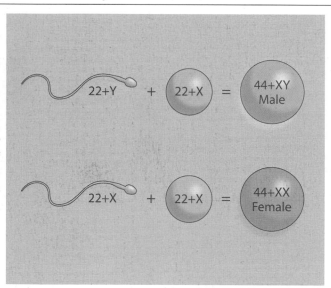

22+Y + 22+X = 44+XY Male

22+X + 22+X = 44+XX Female

- The gender of your baby is determined by the sperm.

- Each sperm carries twenty-two chromosomes and then contributes either an extra Y or an extra X.

- Each egg only has an X chromosome to contribute so the father determines the sex of the baby.

- If he contributes a Y, you will have a boy; if the X is contributed, you will have a girl.

### Twins and More

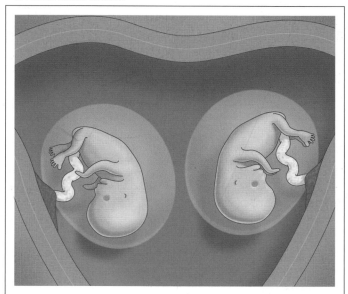

- Twins can be formed either from two of the mother's eggs fertilized separately from two different sperm, or from one egg that divides into two pairs that are genetically identical.

- Triplets and other multiples are nearly always formed when the mother releases several eggs.

- Multiples are more likely to happen to mothers over thirty, those with a family history of twins, and those who have had previous pregnancies.

If you are expecting twins, they can be formed in various ways. One is with two separate eggs and two sperm, known as dizygotic twins or fraternal twins. These twins will have the same genetics as two siblings born at different times. The twins will have separate sacs and placentas. Monozygotic or identical twins are formed when one fertilized egg divides around four to eight days after fertilization. Identical twins will have exactly the same genetic makeup. As you explore questions about your own baby's genetic makeup, you may want to ask your care provider about the tests available.

**ZOOM**

If you will be 35 when your baby is born or you have a history of genetic disorders in your family, you may be referred by your doctor or midwife to a genetic counselor. You will be asked questions about your health status and age, and the health histories and ethnicity of both families. Counselors provide information about potential genetic disorders and a list of options for testing.

## Some Inherited Traits

- Hair color, amount, and texture
- Eye color
- Body structure such as height
- Dimples
- Tongue curling
- Attached/unattached ear lobes

### Baby's Physical Attributes

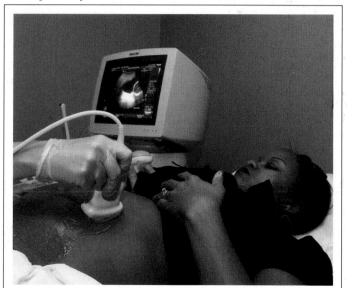

- One of the most exciting things about having a baby is trying to imagine what he or she will look like.

- You each bring a host of your own specific genes that will determine every trait of your baby.

- Will he have his father's nose or his mother's eyes? Will he have his grandmother's red hair?

- It is important for some parents to know the sex of their baby, while others would prefer to be surprised.

PRENATAL TESTING

49

# THE QUAD TEST

## The quad test is one option for parents to screen for Down syndrome and spina bifida

One of the most commonly performed screening tools for genetic problems is known as the alpha-fetoprotein (AFP) Test. The AFP is a prenatal test that screens for genetic disorders such as spina bifida and Down syndrome. It can also be used to screen for defects in the baby's abdominal wall, esophagus, and urinary tract.

If you opt to have this test done, a small vial of blood will be drawn at your care provider's office between your fifteenth and twentieth weeks of pregnancy. The sample will be sent to a lab and results take about a week. Levels of certain hormones in your blood are compared to proteins that are secreted by your baby's liver.

### Quad Screen Up Close

- Screening tool for Down syndrome and spina bifida

- Tests markers in mother's blood

- Offered between fifteen and twenty weeks of pregnancy

- Results available in one week.

- If results show increased risk, referral for amniocentesis

*Choices*

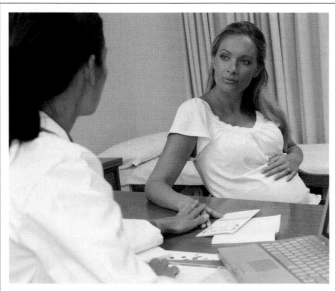

- It is common for your care provider to offer you the AFP as a screening tool in the early part of your pregnancy.

- Some mothers choose to have it done for various reasons.

- However, mothers often forget that just because their doctor offers a test does not mean they have to have it done.

In some cases, your care provider may suggest comparing your hormones to several of the baby's hormones. A Quad screen compares your hormones to the fetal protein produced in the baby's liver. Hormones examined in this screen include hCG, estriol and inhibin, which are all secreted by the placenta.

It is important to remember that the AFP does not have the ability to diagnose your baby's health condition. It merely measures the statistical likelihood of having a baby with genetic problems.

## AFP Is Right for You If:

- you have a family history of genetic problems.
- you have a previous child with genetic problems.
- you are thirty-five or older.

*Discussion*

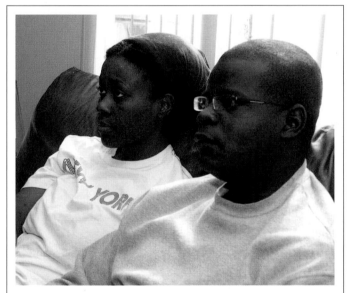

- Prenatal testing during early pregnancy can be stressful for both parents.

- Remember that your care provider or a genetic counselor will be able to answer any of your questions when it comes to results.

- You may decide to go to these appointments together so that you can talk with your care provider about any questions you may have.

- As with any and all medical tests, you have the option to consider them or not.

# THE USES OF ULTRASOUND

## Nearly all pregnant mothers have at least one ultrasound during the course of their pregnancies

Ultrasound is all about sound waves. Your care provider or a sonographer uses a handheld device called a transducer that transmits high-frequency sound waves through your abdomen. When those sound waves reach an object (in this case your baby), an "echo" is created, where the waves bounce back, showing up as an image on the screen.

A transvaginal ultrasound is used in the first trimester as early as five and a half weeks gestation to confirm your pregnancy and determine gestational age. In your second trimester, an ultrasound can look at your baby's development or serve as a follow-up to other prenatal tests. Late in pregnancy your provider may use ultrasound to determine your baby's position or

KNACK PREGNANCY GUIDE

### Ultrasound Up Close

- Confirms pregnancy

- Confirms gestational age

- Used as screening tool for genetic problems or defects

- Tests for baby's health and growth

- Estimates weight of baby

- Used in electronic fetal monitoring

## Ultrasound

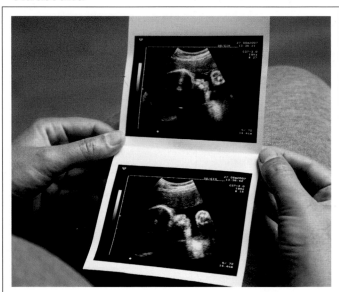

- Ultrasound can help your care provider look at your baby's size and development throughout pregnancy.

- It is also used to examine the location of the placenta and the amount of amniotic fluid.

- Ultrasound may be used to confirm whether or not the mother may have had a miscarriage.

- It is also plays an important role in other prenatal tests such as the NFT and amniocentesis.

to check the baby's lungs for maturity. Most mothers have at least one ultrasound during pregnancy.

Estimating baby's weight via ultrasound is not an exact science. It takes into account head, abdominal, and thigh (femur) measurements to arrive at an estimated weight of your baby. These measurements are occasionally quite accurate, but other times they're not. Any weight estimation by ultrasound can be as much as a pound or more off your baby's actual weight. Often your care provider can more accurately estimate your baby's size by examining your belly.

## Ultrasound in 3-D/4-D

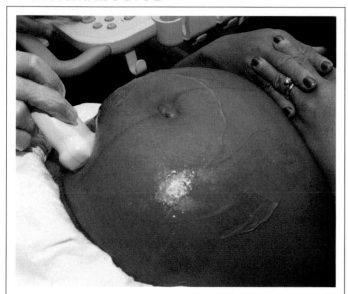

- Your care provider may recommend 3-D or 4-D ultrasound late in your first trimester or early in your second trimester to confirm your baby's well-being.

- The 3-D ultrasound transducer takes a series of images. The computer then translates those images so that they can be seen as three-dimensional images. Four-dimensional images are available as some 3-D scanners can trace the baby's movement.

- The FDA recommends that ultrasound be used for diagnostic and screening purposes only.

## Ultrasound Joys

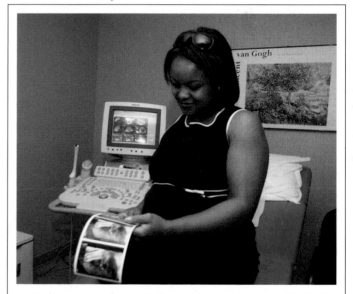

- Mothers report that one of the most enjoyable parts of their pregnancy is hearing the baby's heartbeat.

- Another highlight is getting a glimpse of your baby during a routine ultrasound.

- You would not be the first mother to notice that the use of ultrasound brings you closer to your baby.

- Just bear in mind that less is more when it comes to ultrasound.

# THE FIRST TRIMESTER SCREENING

## The first trimester screening (or triple screen) includes a blood test, ultrasound, and the nuchal fold translucency test

A newer concept in prenatal testing involves combining several screening tools to check for potential genetic problems. One is called the first trimester screen and includes maternal blood tests and an ultrasound known as the nuchal fold translucency (NFT). The NFT measures the space in the tissue located in the nuchal fold at the back of your baby's neck.

The measurement is combined with the gestational age of the baby (based on a crown-to-rump measurement) and the mother's age to determine the statistical likelihood of carrying a baby with Down syndrome.

This three-part test is becoming more popular as a screening tool because it is non-invasive. The first trimester screen

*First Trimester Screen*

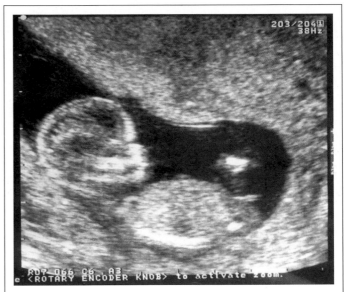

### First Trimester Screening Test Up Close

- Screening tool for Down syndrome
- Offered between eleven and fourteen weeks of pregnancy
- Uses ultrasound to measure folds in baby's neck
- Two chemicals are tested in the mother's blood
- Combines ultrasound with mother's age
- May be referred for diagnostic tests if results are higher than normal

- The ultrasound measurement of the nuchal fold is considered to be a "soft marker" for Down syndrome.

- The other two chromosomal problems that can be screened in this test are trisomy 13 and trisomy 18.

- Some care providers might recommend following up with amniocentesis if there are concerns with the first trimester screen.

- Remember it is always your decision whether or not to agree to more invasive testing.

also has an accuracy of roughly 78 percent in detecting a baby with Down syndrome, versus about 70 percent with simply utilizing the NFT alone.

Keep in mind that this screening test is not able to provide information to parents about other birth defects. Since it is still considered to be a screening test and not diagnostic in nature, your care provider may recommend further testing if there are concerns with your test results.

## ZOOM

A common fear for a pregnant mother is finding out that her baby is not healthy. If you discover your baby has special needs, be sure to seek out resources from your pediatrician, counselors, and support groups for parents who have children with special needs. Many states and government programs have funding for early intervention for your child's physical and intellectual development.

*Dealing with the Facts*

Risk of Down Syndrome by Mother's Age

- 20 years     1 in 1,667
- 25 years     1 in 1,300
- 30 years     1 in 950
- 35 years     1 in 365
- 40 years     1 in 100
- 45 years     1 in 30

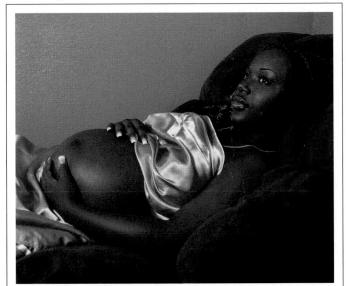

- Sometimes all of the facts and figures and statistics can seem overwhelming to new parents.

- While concerns are normal, keep in mind that nearly all tests come back normal.

- You have a significantly higher chance that everything will be perfect and your baby will be healthy.

- Remember that thinking through your decisions and consulting with your care provider at your earliest opportunity can be reassuring.

# AMNIOCENTESIS
## Amniocentesis has an accuracy rate of over 99 percent in detecting genetic problems in pregnancy

Used during pregnancy for nearly forty years, amniocentesis is the definitive test for genetic defects during pregnancy. In fact, this test can diagnose genetic problems such as Down syndrome, Tay-Sachs, spina bifida, and hemophilia. If you are having your baby tested for genetic problems, you can also find out your baby's gender. Sometimes if your provider is

recommending an early induction or a cesarean before your due date, amniocentesis is used late in pregnancy to confirm your baby's lung maturity.

Once a routine test on mothers over thirty-five, now amniocentesis is recommended as a follow-up to screening tests such as the first trimester screening test and quad screen.

### Amniocentesis Up Close

- Follow-up to screening tests such as AFP, NFT

- Diagnostic test for genetic problems

- Performed between sixteen and eighteen weeks of pregnancy

- Tests for fetal lung maturity near term

### Amniocentesis and Ultrasound

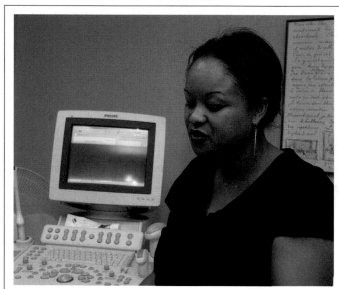

- Ultrasound is a vital component to having an amniocentesis.

- Your care provider will be using the ultrasound transducer to know exactly the location of your baby and your placenta.

- Using the needle, he or she will place the amniocentesis needle in a pocket of amniotic fluid in order to get a small sample.

- That sample is then used to diagnose the health of your baby.

Amniocentesis may be recommended if you already have a child with chromosomal defects or you have a family history of genetic problems. Amniocentesis is performed between fifteen and eighteen weeks. Using ultrasound as a guide, your care provider removes one ounce of amniotic fluid using a needle that is inserted through your abdomen and into your uterus. Final results are available in about two weeks.

Amniocentesis is not risk-free. Complications may occur, although recent improvements in ultrasound and the use of an experienced perinatologist will reduce the risks.

## ZOOM

A brand-new test that detects even the tiniest levels of the baby's DNA in the mother's blood may soon be available to the public. This test may be as accurate as amniocentesis to detect Down syndrome, but without the risk. California researchers believe the test could potentially be used as early as five weeks into a pregnancy.

## Some Genetic Problems Diagnosed by Amniocentesis

- Down syndrome
- Trisomy 18
- Tay-Sachs
- Spina bifida (secondarily)
- Cystic fibrosis
- Sickle cell disease
- Huntington's disease
- Hemophilia
- Muscular dystrophy
- And many more

## The Procedure

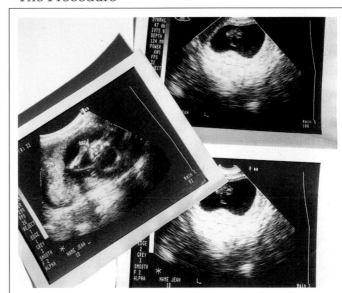

- Since more women are waiting until they are older to have children, it is likely that more prenatal testing, including the use of amnio, is increasing.

- Since amnio requires more expertise and is more invasive, you may be required to have the test done in a different facility than where you plan to give birth.

- It is not unusual to have some discomfort or slight pain after the procedure.

- Check with your care provider to see if you should rest or not return to work after having an amnio.

PRENATAL TESTING

# WHAT ABOUT TEST RESULTS?

## Parents should consider all of the choices they would make based on prenatal test results

Deciding whether or not to have prenatal testing done in the first place is a big decision. The domino effect that occurs when one prenatal test leads to another in early pregnancy is all too common. Waiting for test results (which can take weeks) is difficult. Then what to do with the results can also be a source of stress. Now what do you do if the test is inconclusive? What if your care provider then recommends more invasive testing? Parents might wonder if any of the screening or diagnostic tests could be wrong. How do you decide? The answer is anything but black-and-white.

This is a time when you can and should rely heavily on your care provider's expertise in terms of interpreting the test

### Thoughts

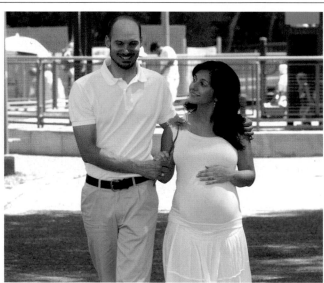

- One question to consider when making decisions about prenatal testing is "How would it help us to know more about our baby?"

- In some cases, having information about your baby's health can give you the time you need to pre-pare, both emotionally and mentally.

- Sometimes having too much information can be the cause of additional stress for parents.

- Think about where you both might be prior to hav-ing tests done.

### Opinions

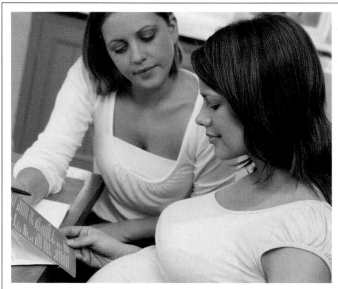

- Sometimes the opinions of others, such as friends and family, are helpful in making decisions such as whether or not to do prenatal testing.

- At other times the opinions of friends only serve to confuse you more.

- What might be right for other people in your life may not be the best gauge for your own decision-making.

- Be sure to thank your friends and family for their advice, but remember that these decisions are yours to make.

results. Remember that your care provider will have his or her own professional opinion about how you should follow-up with those results, but that may not be what is right for you. For some mothers, getting as much information about the health of their baby through prenatal testing is crucial. You might find that the months of pregnancy give you time and opportunity to research any forms of treatment, surgery, or support.

For other parents, starting the process of testing and getting "statistical probabilities" that would lead them further into more invasive testing might not be the right route to take. They might decide to decline testing altogether. Whether or not you would terminate your pregnancy based on test results is another important decision that will likely affect your choice to do any prenatal testing.

The important thing for parents to remember is that your decisions should be made, first and foremost, based on your own beliefs and your attitudes toward your own pregnancy.

## Instinct

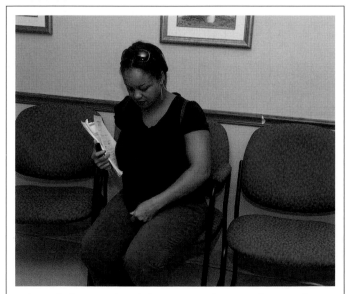

- It can help to get in touch with what you know "in your gut."

- You can think for yourself and, if the situation presents itself, disagree with your care provider.

- In the case of prenatal testing, decisions are, and should remain, deeply personal.

## Support

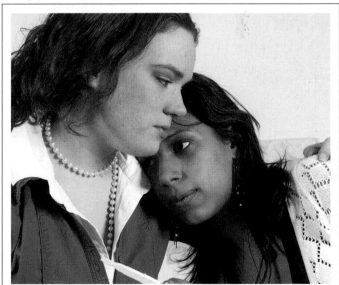

- Start now to reach out for support when you need it.

- It's a skill you will need throughout your pregnancy and beyond in raising your child.

- Who are some of the people you can turn to now? Some of those same people are likely to be the ones you call for support.

- It is no doubt that having a true friend who is a listening ear is worth her weight in gold.

# MAKING DECISIONS

## Choosing a care provider is one of the most important decisions you will make during pregnancy

Even though parents sometimes focus on the wallpaper and the decor of the birthing facility, the place you choose is not nearly as important as choosing the right care provider. A good question to ask yourself in the early part of your pregnancy is "Who do I want supporting and guiding me during pregnancy and birth?" Very often you will have a picture in your mind of who those individuals might be. Perhaps it is an obstetrician. Or you might consider working with a certified nurse-midwife. As you are looking at your options, you may recognize that you are limited in your choices. This could be due to your health-care limitations, insurance, or what is available in your region.

### One or Many?

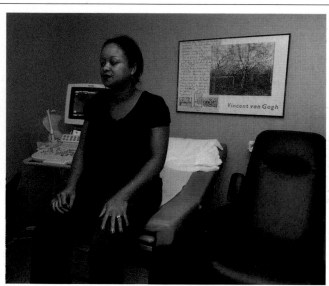

Vincent van Gogh

- The majority of care providers today work in group practices.

- Gone are the days when you could actually select one provider who you knew would be attending your birth.

- You are likely going to need to work with many providers in one practice.

- For that reason, it is important that you schedule prenatal visits with each care provider in the practice to get to know them as much as possible.

### Ask Your Care Provider:

- When would you like me to come to the birth center/hospital?

- What are your recommendations if my water breaks before contractions begin?

- How long after my water breaks would you recommend starting Pitocin?

- What is your philosophy regarding episiotomies?

- What positions for the birth/delivery are you comfortable with?

- How do you feel about natural birth?

If you are not limited in your choice of care provider and you are having difficulty deciding what is best for you, sometimes getting in touch with your feelings about your supportive team is enlightening. Some mothers might write about their vision of who will be helping them through their struggles. You might talk to a trusted friend who has recently given birth. Interviewing specific providers in early pregnancy or beforehand will help you get to know them and to see if your preferences are in line with their practice and philosophy.

## MAKE IT EASY

A childbirth educator I know gives a tip to her students to help them interview care providers: She recommends that they show up early for their scheduled appointments to talk to the new mothers in the waiting room. How was their experience with this provider? Were they satisfied with the care they received? This gives you a consumer's perspective regarding the providers you are interviewing.

*Interviews*

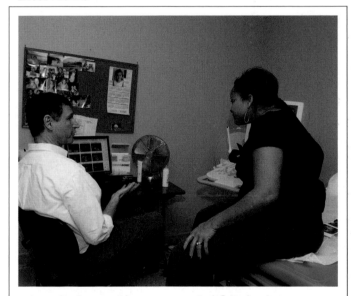

**More Questions to Ask:**

- What is your protocol or routine regarding the following:

  - IVs, continuous monitoring, eating/drinking, walking during labor?

  - hydrotherapy, breaking water, internal monitoring, Pitocin?

- If I choose to use an epidural, when would you recommend I receive it?

- Under what circumstances would you recommend an induction of labor?

- How long after my due date will you wait before inducing labor?

- What non-medical ways of stimulating labor do you recommend?

- Interviewing providers is something that is an important part of planning your birth.

- This is one of the best ways to get your questions answered and feel comfortable with the provider or group you select.

- It definitely takes some extra time out of your busy schedule for interviews.

- However, it will be well worth the time spent interviewing several providers in your area to see which one best meets your needs.

# PERINATOLOGIST

## For a high-risk pregnancy, you may select this type of obstetrician as your care provider

If your pregnancy is considered to be "high-risk," you might be referred to a perinatologist. Perinatologists are obstetricians with an additional three years of training in maternal-fetal medicine, so you might hear these doctors also referred to as maternal-fetal medicine specialists. They will often manage complications with either the mother or the baby or both at any point during pregnancy. Often times the perinatologist works in teaching hospitals in conjunction with a team of specialists who are trained to handle complications that may occur during your pregnancy, labor, or right after you give birth. In some cases you might be referred to a perinatologist for a consultation or to have a specific procedure done

You may choose a perinatologist, or your obstetrician may recommend one, if:

- you are expecting triplets or more.
- you have insulin-dependent gestational diabetes or heart problems, depending on the severity.
- you have recently been diagnosed with or are known to have hypertension.
- you have any infectious diseases such as HIV or hepatitis.
- you have a known or suspected defect with your baby.

### Why See a Perinatologist?

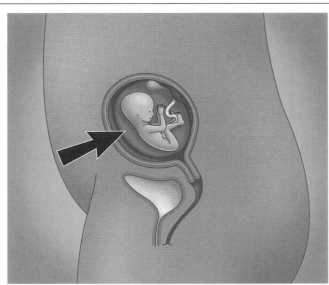

- A common procedure to be referred to a perinatologist for is an amniocentesis.

- You might also see a perinatologist if you have gone past your due date and need to have a biophysical profile.

- These specialists are trained in not only performing these high-tech procedures, but interpreting the results.

- If your pregnancy becomes high-risk and especially when your primary care provider is not able to treat you, these specialists are the ones to help you.

such as an amniocentesis or an in-depth ultrasound if those procedures are not done by your chosen care provider. If you develop pregnancy complications or have existing health problems that an obstetrician or certified nurse-midwife wouldn't be able to manage as well, you may be a candidate for selecting a perinatologist as your primary care provider.

Having a perinatologist who knows the special care you and your baby need may actually put your mind at ease. What is completely unchartered territory for you and your pregnancy will be familiar to a perinatologist.

## Perinatologist Consult

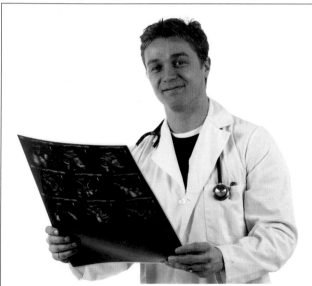

- Sometimes a certified nurse-midwife or obstetrician might recommend a specific test for you.

- You may be referred to a perinatologist for a consultation, even if you do not see her for the remainder of your pregnancy.

- After your procedure is over, your test results will be shared with your primary care provider.

- This is one way that various care providers can work as a team to better meet the individual needs of mothers.

## Perinatologists Up Close

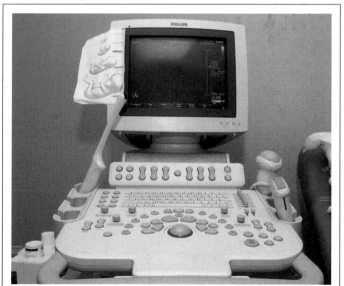

- Perinatologists are trained as obstetricians who work as consultants or primary care providers.

- They have three years of additional training beyond obstetrics and gynecology in maternal-fetal medicine.

- Their specialty is in providing consultation to primary care providers and treating women with high-risk pregnancies.

- Perinatologists often practice in teaching hospitals.

# OB-GYN

## Obstetricians are the most popular choice for pregnant women in the U.S. today

The majority of women in the United States give birth using an obstetrician as their primary attendant. Obstetricians typically handle both obstetrics (delivering babies) and gynecology (women's reproductive health). They are trained as surgeons, so performing a cesarean for an expectant mother or a hysterectomy for a woman in her menopausal years would be familiar territory for today's obstetrician.

One of the downsides to choosing an obstetrician is that since they are such a popular choice, they are often quite busy. You might ask if you can spend extra time getting to know your obstetrician at the end of each prenatal visit. This will give you a perfect opportunity to ask your obstetrician

### An Obstetrician Is Right for You If:

- you plan to give birth in a hospital.
- you need either gynecologic or obstetric care.
- you need to have a cesarean.
- you develop complications and cannot use a midwife.
- you simply prefer an obstetrician.

### Sharing Preferences

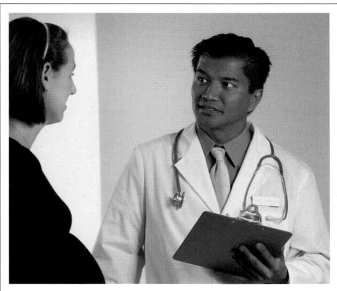

- Spend as much time as possible with your obstetrician during prenatal visits to talk about what your plans, concerns, and expectations are for birth.

- Many mothers write a birth plan to share with their birth team that states their options and preferences.

- Remember that your birth plan is not simply something you write down on paper, but it is also a communication tool.

- The most important thing is to have a discussion with your obstetrician about your preferences prior to giving birth.

64

any questions you may have about his or her philosophy, share your plan for birth, and find out what to expect as your pregnancy progresses.

During labor, obstetricians frequently have a number of patients to attend to. Mothers may not see their obstetrician until late in the pushing stage unless the mother is experiencing complications during labor. The key in choosing the best obstetrician for you is to ask good questions to find who suits your needs the best. The obstetrician's philosophy about pregnancy and birth should match yours.

ZOOM According to the 2002 Listening to Mothers' Survey, about 30 percent of mothers reported that they did not know the care provider who attended their birth or they had only met them briefly before they gave birth.

## Cesarean Birth

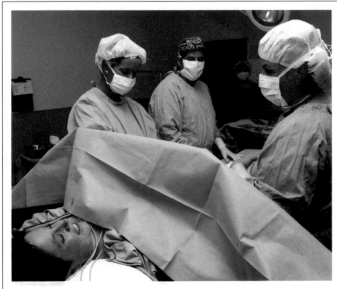

- A few mothers who have health problems early in their pregnancy will know in advance that they need a cesarean rather than a vaginal birth.

- Other mothers learn at the very end of their pregnancy that they would need to schedule a cesarean.

- In some cases, choosing a cesarean will allow you to select a certain care provider if your obstetrician is part of a large group.

- Having this choice gives some mothers a sense of control in planning and the people supporting them during this special event.

## Obstetricians Up Close

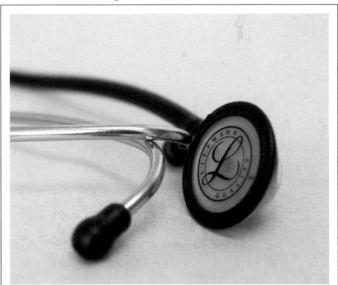

- Obstetricians are typically MDs who are trained as surgeons. They manage both low-risk and high-risk pregnancies.

- OB-GYNs also treat women prior to pregnancy and well past menopause for a range of gynecologic issues. OBs work in hospital settings and often in group practices with other obstetricians.

- They can also serve as backup or provide consultations to certified nurse-midwives.

# CERTIFIED NURSE-MIDWIFE (CNM)

## Certified nurse-midwives offer a personal touch during pregnancy and birth

In many places across the world, certified nurse-midwives (CNM) are the providers of choice for attending births. About 7 percent of women in the U.S. in 2005 used certified nurse-midwives. CNMs are registered nurses who have two years of additional education in the field of midwifery. They can manage low-risk patients and sometimes will have the flexibility to attend births in a hospital or birth center or home births.

Mothers who select a CNM are usually looking for a more natural experience throughout pregnancy and childbirth. CNMs are more likely to incorporate non-medical ways to relieve pain, progress labor, and help mothers find ways to relax.

A CNM Is Right for You If:

- you have a low-risk pregnancy.

- you do not need a cesarean.

- you may want to give birth in an out-of-hospital setting.

- you have a natural philosophy about birth.

- you want more time to spend getting to know your care provider.

### Prenatal Visits

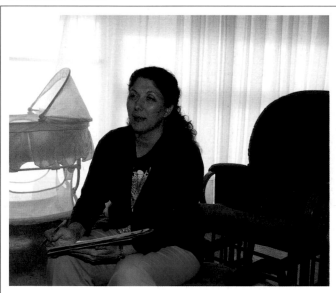

- CNMs may have more flexibility to spend more time getting to know patients during prenatal visits.

- This gives mothers a good opportunity to talk about their needs and concerns during pregnancy and to feel comfortable with their care provider.

- Share with your nurse-midwife the things that are most important to you throughout your pregnancy.

- Keep in mind that babies come at all hours of the day, so you may wait longer to see the nurse-midwife if she is delivering a baby during your appointment.

If you choose a CNM, you most likely want to get to know your care provider during pregnancy and be reassured that you are getting care that is unique to your individual needs.

One disadvantage of selecting a CNM is that you will need to be referred to an obstetrician if you develop complications, whether it is before or during labor. If you need a cesarean or other assisted delivery, an obstetrician will be called in to assist with your care. This is one of the reasons why CNMs are required to have an obstetrician as a backup, in case their patients require surgery or have complications.

## Childbirth

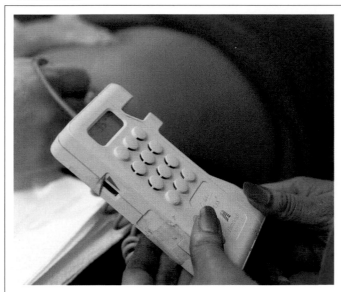

- If you choose a CNM, he or she will likely be with you during the majority of your labor and birth.

- They work as a team with the nurse to record mother's vital signs and progress of labor as well as to monitor the baby's well-being.

- Occasionally the CNM may have other patients in labor, so in that case, having continuous support will not be possible.

- All the more reason to make sure you have adequate support from your partner, family, or birth doula.

## CNMs Up Close

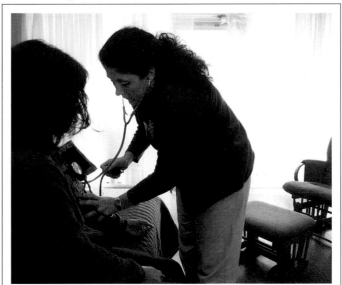

- CNMs are registered nurses with additional training in midwifery.

- They manage only low-risk pregnancies but work with obstetricians as backup when complications occur with mother or baby.

- CNMs practice both in hos-pital and in out-of-hospital settings, such as birthing centers and homebirth.

- CNMs typically have a natural philosophy about birth, but it is recommended that you use our "questions to ask" just to be sure your nurse-midwife is a good fit for you.

# CNM & OBSTETRICIAN
## Obstetricians and CNMs may work together in the same group practice

If you would like to have the advantage of both the medical and non-medical philosophies, you may be interested in a group practice where obstetricians and CNMs work together. Some mothers like the concept of having both types of providers working together and sharing various philosophies with one another. This combined group practice with obstetricians and nurse-midwives can be reassuring to mothers who like the idea that even if complications arise, they would not need to change providers.

These practices can function in different ways. In some obstetrician/CNM groups, the patients would see all of the care providers for prenatal visits, since both doctors and

A Group Practice Is Right for You If:

- you are planning a hospital birth.

- your philosophy is both medical and non-medical.

- you are open to using both types of care providers.

- you have this option available in your area.

*Collaboration*

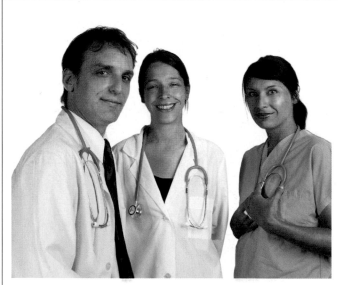

- If you choose a practice with both OBs and CNMs, you can be reassured that they will have an understanding of each other's roles.

- Since they collaborate with one another, you will also find that there is often a sense of mutual respect in this type of practice.

- If a doctor in this practice senses that CNM may be a better fit for the mom, there is no need for a referral.

- A mother may have a sense of safety with a doctor delivering her baby but appreciate that her obstetrician has exposure to other philosophies.

midwives share the time on call equally. In other practices patients can choose either the obstetricians or the midwives to assist them during birth. You also may find group practices where only the doctors are on call to deliver babies. The CNMs in that practice would manage prenatal, postpartum, and gynecologic care for patients; however, they would not be on call to deliver babies.

If you are considering this type of combined practice, be sure you ask how the call time is shared and the roles of each type of care provider.

········· **YELLOW ● LIGHT** ··············

It is not unusual at any stage of pregnancy to discover that you are not seeing eye-to-eye with your provider. If you are not in agreement on several issues in early pregnancy, those issues rarely resolve by forty weeks. If you sense that you need a different provider, go with your instinct. Verify with your health insurance company that you can make the switch before you do. You will be glad you did.

*Sharing Your Plan*

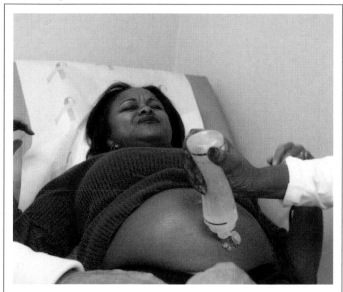

- It will be important to find out if this type of combined practice meets your needs.

- You will still need to share your preferences with all of the care providers in the group.

- Be careful to not assume that every provider in the group has a natural philosophy about pregnancy and birth just because there are CNMs in the group.

- Use your "questions to ask" as a communication tool when you share your plan with all of these providers.

*Easy Transition*

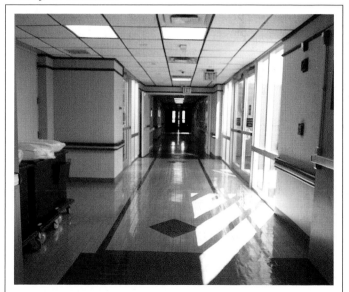

- One distinct benefit when choosing a practice with both care providers is that all parties are in the same practice.

- If you develop a complication and you need to be seen by an obstetrician, your needs will be met without choosing another provider.

- In cases where you were seeing a nurse-midwife but discover that you need to have a cesarean, you will not need to switch to another practice.

- Pregnancy can be stressful. Having the option of a combined practice might be a relief for some mothers.

# BIRTH DOULA
## A doula can be thought of as a "problem-solver" rather than a medical care provider or other support person

Doulas are a recognized member of the birth team, whether mothers plan to give birth in a high-tech setting or at home. Their role is different than that of a primary care provider in that they do not provide medical guidance or perform clinical tasks during pregnancy or labor. Some communities have hospital-based doula programs available, where doulas are provided as a service to expectant families. However, in most cases, families choose to hire their own doula, one who supports the family regardless of where the mother gives birth.

Birth doulas provide support during pregnancy and continuous assistance during birth by making suggestions for comfort, enhancing relaxation, and providing suggestions

### A Birth Doula Is Right for You If:

- you need additional information during your pregnancy.

- you want continuous emotional and physical support during labor.

- you need help with breastfeeding.

- you plan to give birth in any setting.

- you have previously had a difficult labor.

## Meeting Your Doula

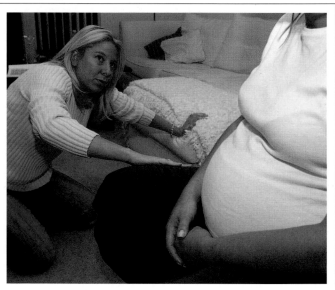

- One of the most important things to look for in a doula is how you both interact and connect with one another.

- You should feel supported in your choices and not pushed in a direction that you are not comfortable in.

- You should, above all, feel listened to, cared for, and understood by the doula you select.

- Using our "questions to ask" will help you discover if the doula you interview is the best one for you.

for labor progress. They assist parents with breastfeeding and postpartum adjustment. They can be thought of as either "problem-solvers" or "encouragers" rather than people who take over your care provider's job or tell you what to do.

Over twenty-five studies have shown that the continuous presence of a doula decreases medical interventions used, shortens the length of labor, increases the likelihood of a vaginal birth, and one of the founders of DONA International, John Kennell, has said, "If a doula was a drug, it would be unethical not to use it."

**ZOOM**

DONA International is the most recognized doula organization in the world today. The founding members of DONA came together in 1992 to recognize the importance of continuous physical and emotional support to the laboring mother and her family. DONA has grown to about 6,500 members and is currently training doulas all over the world. For more information, visit www.dona.org.

## What to Ask

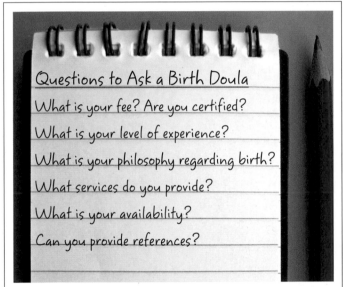

## Birth Doula Up Close

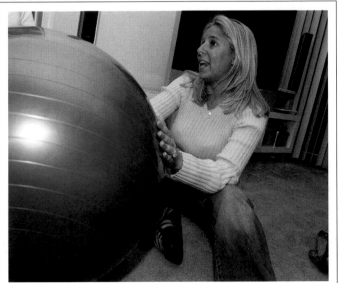

- Birth doulas may offer a range of services including childbirth classes, birth counseling and additional breastfeeding support.

- Costs for birth doula services can vary by region and with the experience level of the doula.

- Doulas who are still in the certification process may offer their services at reduced cost.

- Doulas are often in high demand so if you are considering hiring one, begin interviewing early in your pregnancy.

- Most doulas are certified through recognized organizations such as DONA International. Birth doulas provide only non-medical care to mothers such as emotional support, physical comfort, and assistance in finding information during pregnancy and birth.

- Doulas may work independently, where they are hired by the family or in hospital-based doula programs.

- Birth doulas can work with high- or low-risk clients in hospitals, birth centers or at homebirths.

# MAKING DECISIONS

## From hospital to home birth, choosing your place of birth is as important as choosing your care provider

Part of your early pregnancy planning should be considering where you would like to have your baby. The range of options that are available to women today includes teaching hospitals, community hospitals, free-standing birth centers, in-hospital birth centers, and home birth. Most expectant couples choose hospitals as their place of birth. A smaller percentage will opt to give birth in a birthing center. Only about 1 percent of mothers choose to give birth at home.

Your choice for a place of birth might be limited by your health-care needs and medical insurance as well as what is available in your region. As you start to research the birth settings in your area, you will likely have a greater feeling

### Some Questions to Ask

- What are the policies regarding electronic fetal monitoring?

- Are mothers permitted to eat or drink during labor?

- Can mothers room-in with their babies?

- Does this facility promote breastfeeding?

- How long is the typical stay?

*Taking Tours*

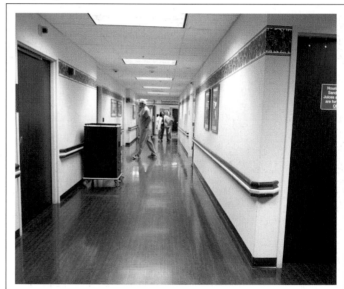

- Make some observations as you walk through tours in each birth setting you are considering.

- Do you see mothers walking around in labor? Do you see staff that are all congregated around the nurses' station or break room talking?

- Is the environment warm and welcoming? Is the staff friendly and open to your questions?

- You might get a sense of how much emotional and physical support you will get in each of these places.

of comfort in one location or another. However, one of the benefits of hiring a birth doula is that no matter what your limitations or comfort level might be, a doula will be able to provide you with continuous support in any birth setting.

As you take tours of various birth settings, picture yourself there. Are options available that are important to you? What is the atmosphere like? Do you feel safe there? It would not be unusual for a mother's labor to slow down simply because she was not feeling safe and secure. Has this place of birth earned a "baby-friendly" label (see Resources)?

## ZOOM

Mothers who choose home birth often do so because they want to have as natural a birth as possible. They want to labor without feeling rushed or pressured into having procedures to speed up labor. Home births allow mothers to eat, drink, change positions, and rest in between contractions as they desire. Labor can happen without the need for medical intervention.

## Comfort

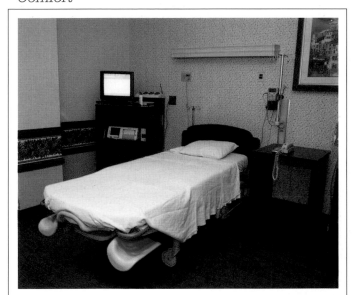

- Not only should the labor room be comfortable to suit the mother's needs, but your chosen place of birth should have some comfortable places for your birth team to rest and take breaks as well.

- If you have family with you, look for areas where they can comfortably wait.

- Find out what options they might have for food and beverages. Some hospitals will provide meals for fathers for an added cost.

- Some hospitals may have several options such as cafeterias or coffee shops.

## Some Steps for Baby-Friendly Hospitals

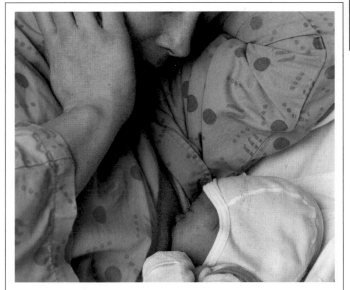

- Maintain a breastfeeding policy; train all health care staff in breastfeeding skills.

- Inform women about benefits and management of breastfeeding and initiate breastfeeding within one hour of birth. Show mothers how to maintain lactation even when separated from babies. Give infants only breast milk unless medically indicated.

- Practice rooming-in and encourage unrestricted breastfeeding. Give no pacifiers or artificial nipples to breastfeeding mothers. Provide support and referrals on discharge.

# TEACHING HOSPITAL

## A teaching hospital is a common choice for mothers at high-risk or with special needs

If you have a preexisting condition or a pregnancy complication that affects you or your baby, you may be choosing a large teaching hospital as your place of birth. Some mothers seek out teaching hospitals because they have teams of experts or specialists who are more familiar with high-risk conditions. If you know that your baby will need to be attended by experts immediately after birth, a teaching hospital will often be the best choice.

Teaching hospitals will have more people participating in the birth process. Not only would you have your chosen care provider, such as a perinatologist or obstetrician, attending to you but you will see residents and medical students on

A Teaching Hospital Is Right for You If:

- you have a high-risk pregnancy.
- you have a preexisting health problem.
- your baby needs specific medical attention/surgery.
- you have unique needs regarding pregnancy.
- you are okay being cared for by medical students and residents.

### Philosophy

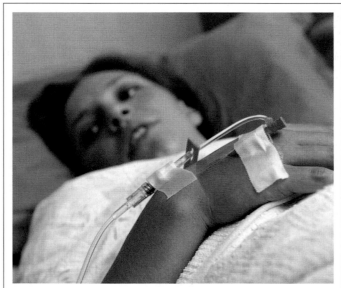

- Because they cater to women who have complications, teaching hospitals will likely have stricter protocols than other birth settings.

- Some of those protocols might include continuous electronic fetal monitoring and restricting mother's fluid intake to ice chips.

- For mothers and babies who need medical interventions, these stricter guidelines are important.

- However, giving birth in a teaching hospital can be a more challenging environment for a low-risk mother who wants to have a natural experience.

the labor and delivery floor as well. What this translates to for the laboring mother is that she will often have multiple people involved in her care, performing vital signs, starting IVs, putting in an epidural, and checking her dilation in labor.

Because the teaching hospital caters to mothers who are high-risk, it is more likely to find that your care will more likely include IVs, continuous monitoring, and eating only ice chips during labor. For those reasons, a teaching hospital will be a more challenging environment for the mother who is seeking a natural childbirth.

**ZOOM**

One little-known fact about teaching hospitals is that because they have specialists on staff, there is a wealth of knowledge and experience for unique situations. For example, if you are expecting multiples or have a breech baby and you are interested in having a vaginal birth, you may be more likely to find a physician able to meet your needs.

## Environment

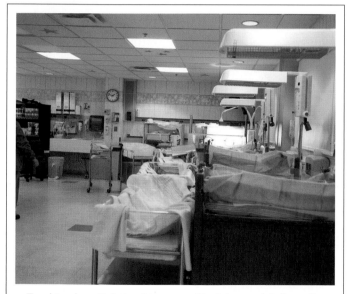

- Teaching hospitals tend to have a lot of technological bells and whistles for mothers and babies.

- High-tech ultrasound equipment, central monitoring systems, and specialized neo-natal intensive care units (NICU) are part of the landscape.

- The labor and delivery floor will be filled with medical students and residents who are busy perfecting their clinical skills.

- You will likely have a team of care providers attending to you during your labor and birth.

## Labor Room

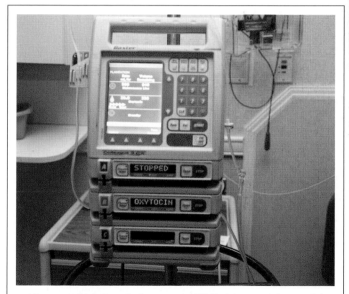

- Many teaching hospitals have renovated their labor rooms to offer a warmer and more inviting environment.

- However, because teaching hospitals house primarily high-risk mothers, it is harder to find options that you might see in other settings such as Jacuzzi tubs.

- While it is certainly possible to have a natural childbirth in a teaching hospital, mothers typically don't choose this location for that reason.

- Should you have any questions about what options are available at your place of birth, check with your care provider or ask on the tour.

# COMMUNITY HOSPITAL

## Many women choose their hometown hospitals because they are convenient to where they live

For many mothers, choosing the local hospital in their hometown is the simplest choice. As expectant parents, you might prefer to get to your birth place quickly in labor and choose a location closer to home, since driving long distances during labor can be stressful. Choosing the community hospital in your area might feel like the most logical choice if you have established relationships with care providers in the past, or your chosen care provider has privileges at this hospital. Perhaps this hospital is where your friends and neighbors have chosen to give birth to their babies. If you live in a rural area, your choices may also be limited to the local hospital.

Options in community hospitals vary greatly. Some

### A Community Hospital Is Right for You If:

- you want to stay in your local community to give birth.

- your community hospital has the options you prefer.

- your community hospital has options your baby needs.

- your chosen care provider has privileges at this location.

*Philosophy*

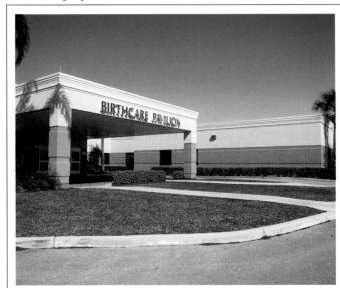

- View your hospital's philosophy by taking a tour, talking to your care provider, and talking to parents who have given birth there.

- If you are planning a VBAC (vaginal birth after a cesarean) but you find that your local community hospital does not allow VBACs, you will need to choose a different setting where a trial of labor is possible.

- Check in with your care provider about any specific anesthesia requests.

- Be wary of birth plans found on the Internet, as they can be misleading.

community hospitals have flexible protocols and adapt easily to mothers who have different needs and concerns. For example, your local hospital may have things like portable monitors and tubs for laboring in. Some hospitals may carry extra birthing balls for laboring mothers to use during labor. Or you might find on the other hand that your community hospital is a bit more traditional in their approach to childbirth. The best thing to do is take a tour of your community hospital(s) or talk to your care provider to see what options are available, and if those options suit your needs.

**ZOOM**

Many hospitals today have labor beds with multiple buttons that adjust the head and foot of the bed and even provide more lumbar support. Some will turn the TV on or off and adjust the volume. There is also an alert button on the bed panel to call your nurse. Ask your labor nurse for a tutorial on how to use the labor bed and its various gadgets when you arrive during labor.

## Environment

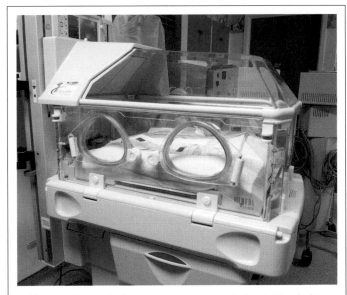

- The good news is that many hospitals today pay attention to what consumers ask for when it comes to birth.

- The birthing environment has changed drastically from the days when fathers were not allowed in the room to witness the birth of their babies.

- Instead of whisking babies off to the nursery, most hospitals allow mothers to "room-in" with their babies.

- Compared to mothers in the past who were often alone, many hospitals are open to having several support people in the room to assist mothers.

## Labor Room

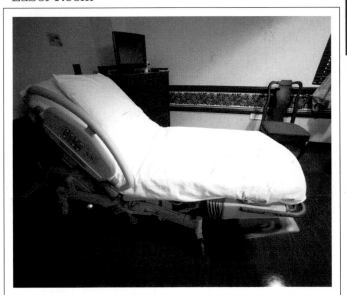

- A hospital labor room might include beautiful hardwood floors and a pull-out sofa for fathers to sleep in or a tiny room with a few chairs for support people.

- Some labor tools, such as your birth ball, can serve as a comfortable seat when not being used by moms.

- You can also bring familiar things from home such as your own robe or pillows.

- Comfort is important, but don't forget that it's truly the people supporting you that will make the biggest difference in your labor.

# IN-HOSPITAL BIRTH CENTER

## The in-hospital birth center combines a homelike atmosphere with proximity to the labor and delivery floor

Some expectant mothers may choose to have their baby in a birth center that is located within a hospital setting. An in-hospital birth center may consist of several birthing rooms or suites that are adjacent to or in a different wing of the hospital, in close proximity to the labor and delivery floor and the operating rooms.

Mothers who choose this option are typically planning to use a variety of non-medical pain relief measures instead of more traditional options for pain medication. These centers may provide birthing tubs, squatting bars, birth balls, birthing chairs, and a host of other comfort measures for mothers to use during labor. They often allow the mother to eat lightly

An In-Hospital Birth Center Is Right for You If:

- you have a low-risk pregnancy.
- you plan to have a natural childbirth.
- you want non-medical options for pain and labor progress.
- you want to have proximity to a hospital.
- you plan to use a CNM.

*Philosophy*

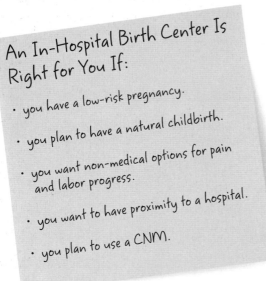

- In-hospital birth centers have a bent toward recognizing the natural process of labor.

- While they recognize the need for medical assistance, it is assumed that mothers will not need those hospital procedures.

- If you are thinking of having an epidural, the philosophy of an in-hospital birth center might not align well with your own philosophy.

- However, one advantage of an in-hospital birth center is that there is a close proximity to medical interventions should your plans change.

and drink fluids as she desires. Fetal monitoring is often done by checking the baby's heartbeat periodically with a hand-held doppler, which is similar to what many providers use during a mother's prenatal visit. Many in-hospital birth centers are staffed by certified nurse-midwives as well as labor and delivery nurses.

One advantage of an in-hospital birth center is the close proximity to the hospital should the mother develop a complication. If a mother's plans change, she can easily be transferred to the main part of the hospital.

## Environment

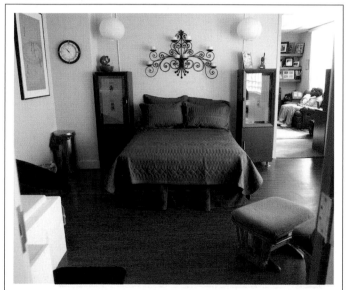

- You will likely see mothers walking around during labor and many birth centers include tubs or showers for hydrotherapy.

- CNMs and nurses will monitor your baby intermittently or check periodically with a Doppler ultrasound.

- Sometimes mothers will be able to eat light foods and/or drink clear fluids.

- Be sure to check with the local in-hospital birth centers in your area since routines and options can vary.

## Labor Room

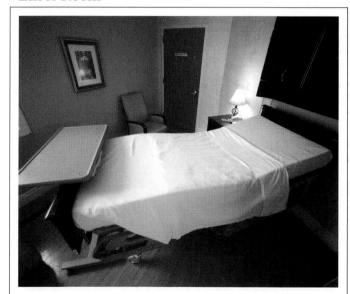

- Most in-hospital birth centers have birthing suites that look a lot like your bedroom at home.

- Some may have a typical hospital bed with a few extra chairs for support people.

- Others will have cozy furniture for guests and a double bed for mothers to use during labor and after birth.

- The medical equipment is accessible in each room but stored away, since staff will not likely need to use it.

# FREE-STANDING BIRTH CENTER

## Free-standing birth centers are a popular choice for mothers planning to have a natural childbirth

A free-standing birth center is one that is truly separate from the hospital, run by certified nurse-midwives, and often includes non-medical pain relief options, such as birthing tubs. Some are owned and operated privately, while others may be owned by a hospital, physician's practice or medical institution. All free-standing birth centers have a transfer hospital nearby where mothers and babies can go should complications arise during or immediately after birth.

One of the biggest draws to a free-standing birth center is the freedom mothers have throughout labor. Mothers are able to eat and hydrate as they wish. Mothers can move and change positions for comfort at any stage in labor. Many

### A Free-standing Birth Center Is Right for You If:

- you have a low-risk pregnancy.
- you plan to use a CNM.
- you plan to have a natural childbirth.
- you want non-medical options for pain and labor progress.
- you want to go home shortly after birth.

*Philosophy*

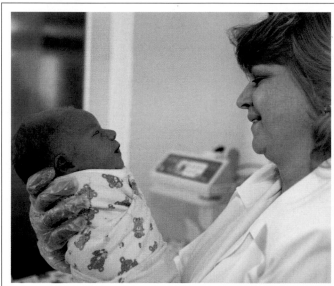

- A free-standing birth center has a philosophy that pregnancy and birth are normal and healthy events.

- Because birth is viewed as a normal event, in most cases it should not be a medical intervention.

- There is a sense at a birth center that with enough support and patience, most mothers can achieve a natural birth.

- If this philosophy aligns with your own, then choosing to give birth in a freestanding birth center might be for you.

mothers also enjoy being able to have an unlimited number of friends or family to support them. Typically parents would leave a birth center about four to eight hours after giving birth, which is either a plus or a minus for mothers, depending on their own preferences.

Research shows that about 10 to 12 percent of mothers will need to be transferred from a free-standing birth center to the closest hospital at some point during labor. One of the most common reasons for a transfer is a slow or non-progressing labor and/or the need for pain medication.

## Environment

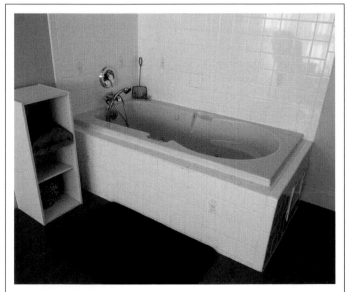

- The environment at free-standing birth centers tends to be more peaceful and private as compared to a hospital environment.

- Since birth is treated like a normal event, mothers do not have to stick to clear fluids and can eat or drink whatever they wish.

- It is not unusual to find mothers laboring and giving birth in a tub in a freestanding birth center.

- Since interventions are rare, mothers will be ready to go home on average six hours after giving birth.

## Labor Room

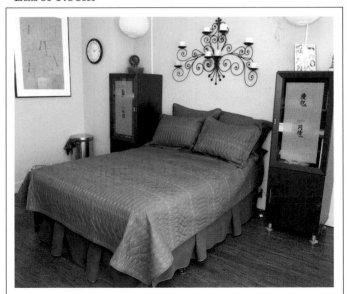

- Labor rooms in a free-standing birth center are designed to look just like yours at home, except maybe less cluttered.

- A double or queen bed is standard and many have birthing chairs, birthing balls, and CD players.

- Moms will be moving about freely during labor and using a variety of positions to keep labor progressing and reduce pain.

- This is one of the birth settings where the mothers may be less likely to give birth in the bed than anywhere else.

# PRECIPITOUS BIRTH

## Parents sometimes find out that baby has other plans when it comes to birth location

A precipitous birth is just a medical term for a labor that lasts three hours or less from start to finish. While precipitous labors are not predictable, most often these rare, but rapid labors will happen with a subsequent birth. You are also more likely to have another precipitous labor if you have already had one before.

So how will you know if this type of labor is happening to you? One way you can tell is that the intensity of labor builds very quickly. Your contractions may even start out at five minutes apart rather than fifteen minutes apart! You might even notice pressure in your rectum not too long after contractions have started.

### Call 911

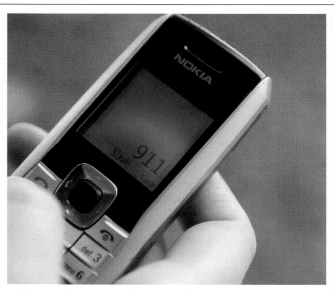

- If you are not sure you have time to get to your place of birth, you don't have to try to do everything by yourselves.

- Pick up the phone and dial 911.

- The emergency operators are trained to talk you through what to do before the EMTs arrive.

- The most important thing to do is to stay calm and remind yourselves that your baby is simply coming in a different place than you planned.

### What You Need

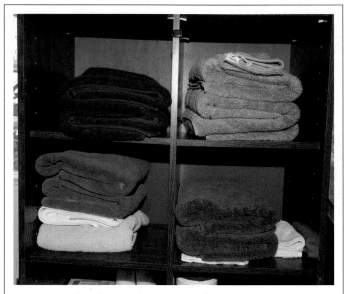

- Surprisingly, a healthy baby only needs two things in the first few moments of life: to have a clear airway and to be kept warm.

- Right after the baby is born, you can use a clean towel or any clean item of clothing you have handy to cover baby and mother.

- Be sure to put baby skin-to-skin on the mother's chest and cover them both with a clean towel since mom's body is the warmest place for baby.

- If baby is not crying, you can rub her back or her feet vigorously—but they do not like their feet tickled.

The big question now is what should you do? If you are feeling a strong urge to bear down or you can feel your baby's head and you live thirty minutes from the hospital, it may be safer to stay home and call 911. They will talk you through what to do if your baby is coming quickly.

Remember that precipitous labors are rare. It is much more likely that your labor will last for twenty hours as compared to two hours. Knowing what to do if your labor is faster than you expected will help you stay calm amidst the mayhem.

## Baby Is Here!

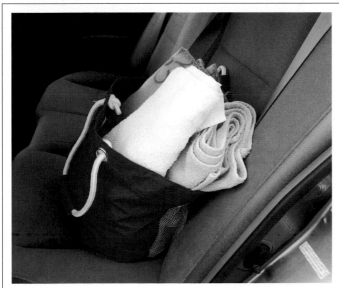

- Parents who have an unplanned home birth might feel like a deer in headlights for the first few days.

- If you had planned to give birth in the hospital you might be in denial at first that things did not go as planned.

- It is also not unusual for mothers to feel responsible that they missed some signs telling them when to leave for their place of birth.

- Bear in mind that usually these babies that come quickly seem to roll with the changes better than mom and dad.

### Tips for Baby Birthing

- Remain calm.

- Call 911 and unlock the front door.

- Grab clean towels.

- Wash your hands if time allows.

- Instruct Mom to pant instead of push if possible.

- Cover baby with clean towels on mom's chest.

- Rub baby's back or feet to stimulate breathing (if needed).

- Wait for help to arrive and further instructions.

# MAKING DECISIONS

## Options for the environment, size, and content of childbirth classes vary widely today

Part of your preparation for birth includes taking a childbirth class. As you explore your options, there are many things to keep in mind. Classes that have eight or more couples participating will feel much more impersonal. Look for classes with no more than four to six couples so that you have ample time to ask questions and get to know your childbirth educator.

Be sure that you find out if the educator's philosophy about birth matches yours before you sign up! There is nothing worse than having to filter out what is being taught because you are not in agreement with the instructor. Some classes may focus exclusively on one method versus teaching a variety of methods for pain. You will need a variety of coping tools

### Questions to Ask

- How many couples typically attend?
- Is a particular method taught?
- How much time is provided to practice?
- Is the childbirth educator certified?
- What is the educator's philosophy about birth?
- What does the course content include?
- Are references available?

### Learning Environment

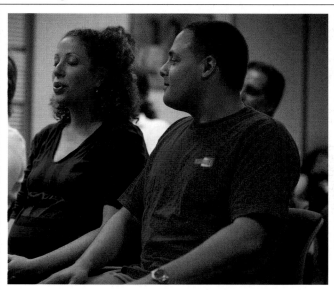

- Do you want to take the class to meet other parents, hear their questions, and enjoy socializing?

- Or do you prefer just getting the information straight from the instructor in a one-on-one learning situation?

- Do you like being in a home environment for class or do you prefer that classes take place where you also plan to give birth?

- Figuring out what you prefer will help you decide which childbirth class is best for you.

rather than just one method. You should also find out how much time the instructor allows for practice of techniques. Parents may not remember much from a class that offers only lecture and no time to practice or review techniques.

Ask about course content and if it includes information about postpartum care and breastfeeding. For some mothers, this is a more challenging time than birth. You might be able to speak with a parent who has finished the childbirth class just to see if the class is right for you.

Years ago nearly all mothers took childbirth preparation classes and learned techniques to cope with pain. Epidurals were used only after other methods failed. Now more mothers plan exclusively for epidurals, sometimes omit childbirth classes altogether, and are often unprepared when the epidural doesn't help or there is a delay in getting one. Remember that preparation is the ticket to knowing your options and what to expect, no matter what happens during your labor!

## Learning Styles

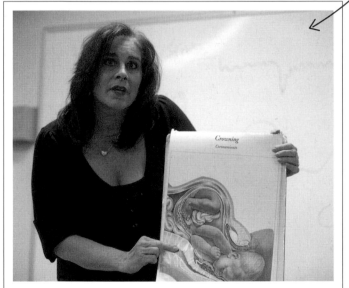

- We do not all learn the same way.

- Some people are visual learners, so they will need photos, videos and plenty of audio-visuals to get the most from classes.

- Some are auditory learners, so they might prefer hearing music in class or working in groups to hear what others have to say.

- And others are kinesthetic or tactile learners who learn by doing things, so they will enjoy lots of hands-on practice. Ideally, your childbirth class offers instruction for all types of learners.

## Instructor Rapport

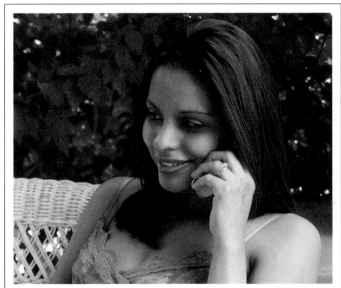

- Did you ever have a teacher who you did not agree with? It was probably hard for you to learn because you didn't trust new information.

- To avoid this in a childbirth class, talk to your childbirth educator on the phone first.

- Is she a good listener? Do you feel she is open to hearing your concerns?

- Rapport with the childbirth educator only improves the experience of taking classes.

# CLASS LOCATION

## Learn more about the two most popular locations for childbirth classes

As you are exploring your options for classes, an important factor to investigate is the location in which the classes are held. Who is the sponsor of the class? Is there any affiliation between the educator and the institution? Sometimes this can have an effect on the flavor of the class as well as the content of what is taught in the course.

Over the last several years, hospital-based classes have shortened the length of their programs. This could mean that parents have a limited amount of time to learn or practice comfort measures. Educators in a hospital program—often labor and delivery nurses—may not have freedom to talk about subjects that might be in conflict with the practices

### Hospital Classes Are Right for You If:

- you plan to use an epidural.

- you have not made up your mind about pain medication.

- you don't mind a class with many participants.

- you prefer a shortened class.

- you want the least expensive class.

*Certification*

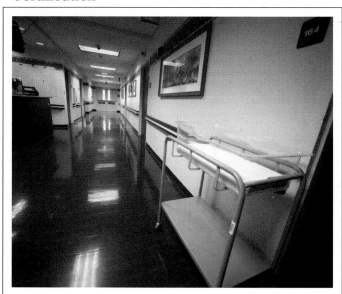

- Not many parents recognize that the certification of the childbirth educator plays a role in the flavor of the class, possibly even more so than the location of the course.

- Find out more about where the educator was certified and what was involved in the certification process.

- Certification should involve a training program, writing a course curriculum and taking a written exam.

- Also find out if part of the certification involved evaluation of a teaching series by an experienced educator.

of medical staff. However, these nurses can present a realistic picture of how various labors may progress. Having a one-on-one conversation with the educator prior to registering for the course will provide answers to your questions. One benefit of taking a class at your local hospital is that the classes are usually the best bargain. Another benefit is that the class often includes a tour of the labor and delivery rooms.

On the other hand, independent educators will have freedom to share new ideas, the latest research findings, and how best to advocate for yourselves as expectant parents.

These courses also tend to be longer and include a comprehensive curriculum. Independent educators may hold the classes in their home or in a comfortable setting such as a birth center.

Regardless of where you take classes, find out if the educator is certified by a recognized organization. If so, you can be assured that she has completed a rigorous program and not only has a knowledge base about current birth issues but also has good teaching skills.

## Word of Mouth

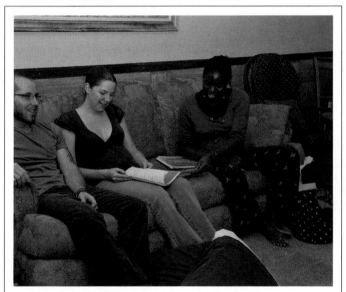

- Chances are high that you'll hear about educators who teach privately by word of mouth rather than finding a listing in the phone book.

- A word-of-mouth referral from a happy customer is often the best recommendation.

- However, it still makes good sense to spend time talking with the educator on the phone prior to registering.

- Don't forget to check with your insurance company to see if it may reimburse you for classes.

### Independent Childbirth Education Is Right for You If:

- you have a more natural philosophy of birth.

- you prefer a small number of participants.

- you want time to practice techniques in class.

- you are interested in a more in-depth course.

- you prefer a more comfortable setting.

- you don't mind spending a bit more for classes.

# THE "NEW" LAMAZE
## Lamaze is no longer about teaching patterned breathing for labor— it now stands for normal birth

The Lamaze method was originally developed in France by Ferdinand Lamaze in 1951. The method consisted of childbirth classes, relaxation and breathing, and support by a trained nurse and the patient's partner. Marjorie Karmel and Elizabeth Bing brought the method to the United States to teach it to as many mothers as possible. In 1960 they formed

ASPO/Lamaze, now known as Lamaze International.

When you hear "Lamaze" now, likely your first thought is "breathing." While learning patterned breathing was a key component to the early Lamaze method, it no longer plays a central role. Instead, the emphasis of education is on the Lamaze philosophy of birth. In a nutshell, Lamaze tries to

### Lamaze Philosophy

- Birth is normal, natural, and healthy.

- The experience of birth profoundly affects women and their families.

- Women's inner wisdom guides them through birth.

- Women's confidence and ability to give birth is either enhanced or diminished by the care provider and place of birth.

- Women have the right to give birth free from routine medical interventions.

- Birth can safely take place in homes, birth centers, or hospitals.

- Childbirth education empowers women to make informed choices in health care, to assume responsibility for their health, and to trust their inner wisdom.

### Comfort Techniques

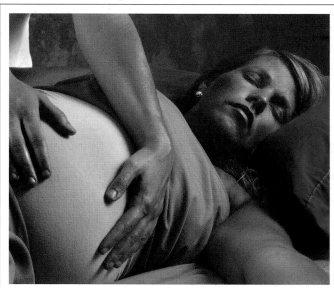

- Not all mothers cope with the pain or challenges in the same way during labor.

- Some might like quiet and darkness; other might prefer the blinds open, lights on, and plenty of visitors.

- Some mothers love to be massaged, while others will not want to be touched.

- Practicing a variety of tools to relieve pain and discomfort is a good strategy for all mothers, regardless of the type of class they attend.

bring attention to the importance of birth in the woman's life, and advocates that parents ought to be given the freedom to choose how and where they want to have a baby.

The Lamaze method recommends a minimum of twelve hours of childbirth classes that cover pregnancy, stages of labor, comfort techniques, role of the partner/father, medications and medical intervention, cesarean birth, breastfeeding, postpartum issues, and parenting the newborn. You can find Lamaze-certified educators at www.lamaze.org.

## Massage in Labor

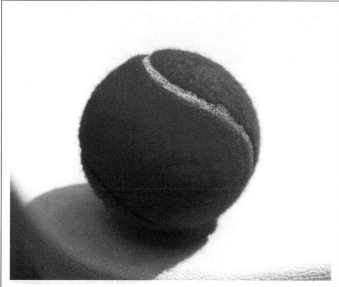

- A good childbirth class includes a review of various massage techniques.

- Some of the best techniques to practice include stroking, kneading, and firm counter-pressure. The use of a tennis ball can help.

- Massage works well to distract mother from the pain by giving her a competing sensation that is pleasurable.

- It also helps to reduce pain by putting pressure directly on painful areas such as the mother's back.

Lamaze Is Right for You If:

- you are on the fence about pain meds.

- you are planning a drug-free labor.

- you have six or more weeks to devote to class.

CHILDBIRTH CLASS

# DRUG-FREE LABOR WITH BRADLEY

## Relaxation and the father's role as birth partner are central themes in the Bradley Method of childbirth

The American Academy of Husband-Coached Childbirth, or Bradley Method, was inspired by obstetrician Robert Bradley, who developed this method in 1947 based on observations he made while watching mammals during labor. He believed that women, like animals, could give birth without medication if they used relaxation and natural abdominal breathing as well

as support from their husband. His findings played a major role in encouraging the father to participate in the birth process. Marjie and Jay Hathaway took his method and founded the American Academy of Husband-Coached Childbirth (AAHCC).

The primary goal of the Bradley Method is "healthy mothers and healthy babies." The method teaches that under most

### Mammals in Labor

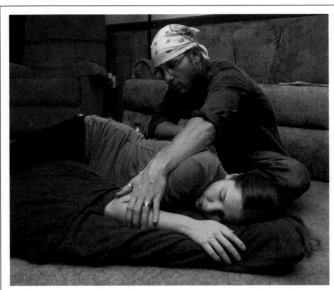

- Robert Bradley came up with his childbirth method by studying mammals in labor.

- Mammals change positions throughout labor. Sometimes they rest on their sides while in labor, and other times, they are up and moving.

- Mammals breathe deeply during contractions to aide the progress of labor. These female mammals labor by instinct and respond to what their bodies tell them to do.

- Dr. Bradley believed that observations of mammals can help humans respond more instinctively to labor.

### Bradley Classes

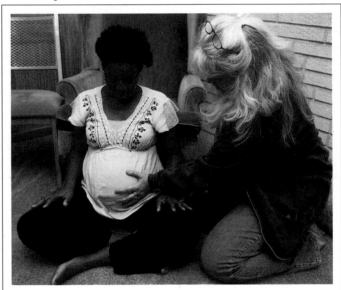

- At the heart of the Bradley method is the role of the father as primary "coach" for labor.

- This method is one of the most in-depth childbirth classes available and includes about twenty-four hours of class time.

- Bradley educators limit the size of their classes to six couples to provide a more intimate learning environment.

- These classes are geared toward mothers and partners who are committed to have a natural childbirth.

circumstances, a drug-free labor is the best way to achieve that goal. In addition to relaxation and natural breathing, the course content focuses on the role of healthy nutrition and other ways to stay low-risk during pregnancy and labor, to avoid complications and medical interventions. The AAHCC reports that 86 percent of the mothers who participate in their program have drug-free, vaginal births.

The AAHCC course is twelve weeks in length and is designed to take place in the final trimester of pregnancy. The size of the class is ideally four to six couples.

## Relaxation Exercises

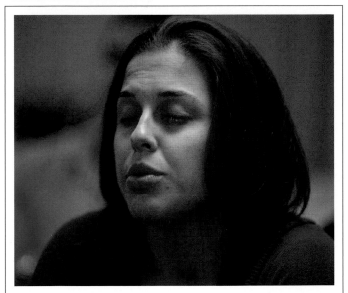

- The focus of the Bradley method for coping with labor is relaxation.

- Mothers are encouraged to relax during and in between contractions as compared to learning a series of patterned breathing techniques.

- A review of relaxation combined with deep abdominal breathing is offered several times throughout the twelve-week course.

- Students are encouraged to practice various techniques with their partners in between classes.

### The Bradley Method Is Right for You If:

- you have a natural philosophy of birth.

- you are committed to a drug-free birth.

- you have a supportive partner.

- you are interested in an in-depth class.

- you have ten to twelve weeks available for classes.

# BIRTH WORKS

## Birth Works International is a newer childbirth education program that emphasizes trusting your body

The Birth Works childbirth concept formally began in 1981 by Cathy Daub, a physical therapist, who wanted to instill in women the knowledge that their bodies already know how to give birth. By 1988 a formal program was developed with the first childbirth educator training. Birth Works does not consider itself to be a "method" course but rather a "process."

Some of the philosophy of Birth Works is based on encouraging a mother to express emotions and become more aware of how her beliefs affect her birth.

Birth Works educators will impart to couples that there is no "right way" to give birth and that each birth is unique. An emphasis is placed on enhancing the environment during

### Philosophy

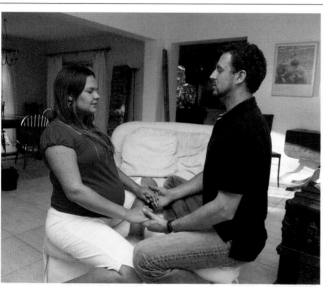

- The philosophy of Birth Works is that a woman does not need to be taught how to give birth.

- Instead, she needs help to recognize that her body already has the knowledge it needs to give birth.

- Birth Works emphasizes that women need to learn to trust in their own inner wisdom.

- This inner wisdom is what will help guide her throughout labor and in making decisions that are right for her.

### Birth Works Classes

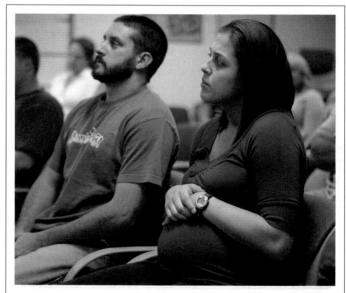

- During the Birth Works class, parents will learn breathing awareness, relaxation and directed breathing as ways of coping with contractions.

- Classes also include a segment on healthy nutrition and exercise for pregnancy.

- Since labor is unpredictable, the course also covers medical procedures and medications.

- Parents also learn about positions for labor, the role of the birth team, the grief process and healing, as well as issues of breastfeeding and postpartum.

labor so that the mother feels safe. The exact location of that birth is up to the woman herself and what she feels is best for her.

Rather than any specific breathing pattern, slow, deep breathing and relaxation are taught during class. Pelvic bodywork is also taught, which enables the mother to identify how her pelvis moves and opens in various positions.

Course length is anywhere from six to ten weeks, and parents are encouraged to begin the class as early in pregnancy as possible.

## Pelvic Bodywork

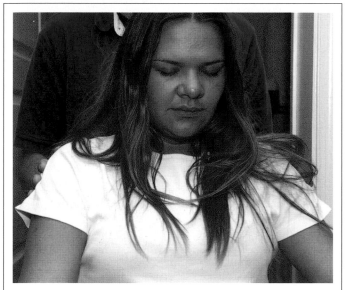

- Birth Works classes stress the importance of technique known as "pelvic bodywork" to prepare mothers for labor.

- Pelvic bodywork includes developing an understanding of how your own pelvis moves and works.

- The instructors remind mothers about the flexibility and softening of the pelvic ligaments and joints.

- Pelvic bodywork helps mothers to feel comfortable with their own bodies and the movements of their pelvis by practicing relaxation and breathing exercises.

It seems that fewer mothers are participating in childbirth classes today. According to the Listening to Mothers Survey from 2002, about 70 percent of first-time mothers took classes. However, a follow-up survey four years later indicated that only about 50 percent of mothers took childbirth classes with their first baby.

Birth Works Is Right for You If:

- you want to explore your emotions during pregnancy.

- you want to learn more about trusting your body.

- you would prefer a class where your choices are respected.

- you have six to ten weeks for classes.

# COPE WITH HYPNOSIS

## The HypnoBirthing Method teaches mothers to use self-hypnosis for coping with labor pain

HypnoBirthing, also known as the Mongan Method, uses relaxation, breathing, and self-hypnosis in its approach to childbirth preparation. The founder, Marie Mongan, is a hypnotherapist and incorporates self-hypnosis techniques in her book, HypnoBirthing, which was written in 1989.

The concept of HypnoBirthing borrows the idea of the fear-tension-pain cycle from Dr. Grantly Dick-Read, one of the first proponents of natural childbirth back in the 1920s. The method teaches expectant mothers that, in the absence of fear and tension, the sensation of pain can be reduced.

Educators will teach you that learning self-hypnosis is not like losing consciousness or being asleep, but closer to a

### HypnoBirthing Method

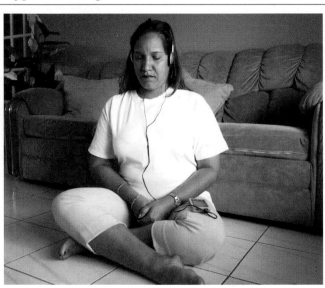

- Marie Mongan's Hypno-Birthing method emphasizes reducing the fear that often accompanies childbirth.

- Parents learn to use self-hypnosis, guided imagery, and breathing techniques to help them give birth without medication.

- She claims that laboring women will be alert and able to participate throughout the birth process.

- Observations of mothers who have used this method indicate that they are not always alert and responsive and often look like they are in a trance.

### Rainbow Relaxation

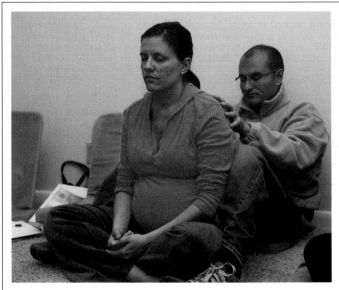

- One of the popular relaxation exercises includes focusing on the image of a rainbow.

- This is one of the many scripted images that HypnoBirthing encourages mothers and their partners to practice before labor.

- The rainbow image involves the birth partner guiding the mother through a series of images incorporating all of the colors of the rainbow.

- Some mothers may enjoy designing their own relaxation or imagery exercise even if you do not choose this childbirth method.

state of daydreaming. Mothers are also told that they will often experience a time distortion while in a hypnotic state.

The course is taught over twelve hours, and mothers and partners learn to use scripted self-hypnosis techniques to work through her fears and challenges during labor and birth. This is strictly a method class and in many ways is not comparable to other childbirth preparation courses. It does not typically include a discussion of medical interventions, cesareans, or recovery after surgery, or of breastfeeding and postpartum issues.

## Laboring with Hypnosis

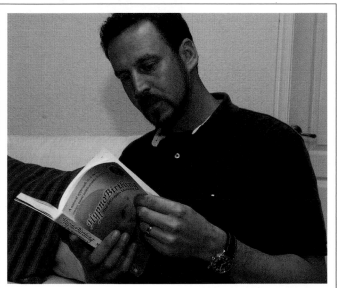

- It is good to let your care providers know as soon as you arrive at your place of birth that you are using hypnosis for labor.

- This could also be part of your written birth plan or discussion with your care provider.

- One of the reasons is that, unlike other methods, HypnoBirthing involves a unique set of birth-related language.

- Since the language used for labor with this method is very different, parents should explain these differences to their care provider.

**HypnoBirthing Is Right for You If:**

- you have a lot of fear going into childbirth.

- you are comfortable with self-hypnosis.

- you prefer a method-style class.

- you plan to take a separate course for breastfeeding.

- you plan to take a separate baby care class.

CHILDBIRTH CLASS

# YOUR FIRST-TRIMESTER CHECKLIST

## Making healthy food decisions and avoiding exposure to chemicals are essential aspects of the first trimester

It is a very good thing that pregnancy takes nine months. There is so much to do in preparation for the baby that it can take every one of those nine months for you to finish everything.

The first trimester is a great time to begin planning, making decisions and getting organized. This would be a perfect time to think more about what you are eating and how to get all of the necessary nutrients in your diet. Since the first trimester is the most sensitive time for your baby's development, avoiding any exposure to harmful substances like alcohol, smoking, and unnecessary medications will be critical.

Some of your first-trimester planning involves interviewing

### First-Trimester Checklist

- Start taking prenatal vitamins and eating healthy foods.

- Avoid exposure to harmful substances (smoking, alcohol, X-rays, unnecessary medications).

- Interview and select providers.

- Take tours and select birthing facility.

- Decide which prenatal tests to take.

- Research childbirth classes.

- Begin reading up on pregnancy issues.

- Interview birth and/or postpartum doula.

### Healthy Nutrition and Vitamins

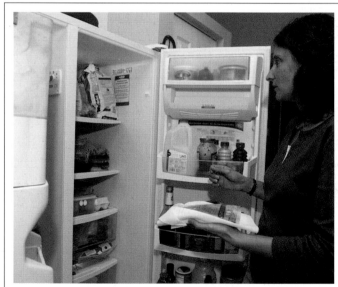

- Start your pregnancy diet out right by taking prenatal vitamins several months prior to getting pregnant, throughout pregnancy, and during breastfeeding.

- Your diet should be an important focus of your first trimester checklist since

this is when your baby's organs are developing.

- Try to eat a variety of proteins, fruits, vegetables, and carbohydrates in your meals and snacks.

care providers. If you are planning to use a birth doula, start looking for one now, since they can book early! You will also be exploring where you feel comfortable having your baby and taking tours at the birthing facilities in your area.

Deciding how to feed your baby is also something most mothers begin to do early in pregnancy. Reading books and scanning Web sites for expectant parents can help you get more information about breastfeeding as well as other aspects of pregnancy and baby care.

## What to Read

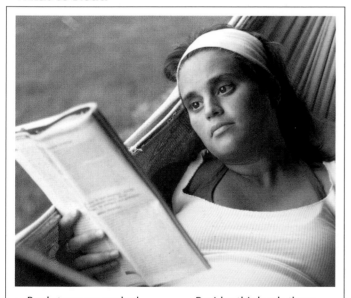

- Bookstores are packed with books on pregnancy nutrition, childbirth, breast-feeding, and methods of parenting your baby.

- Knowing what books are worth reading, as well as who the experts are in this field, can be challenging to a new mother.

- Besides this book, there are some great titles out there that we can recommend that can help prepare you for all aspects of your pregnancy.

- Please refer to the resource section for more information.

## Changes

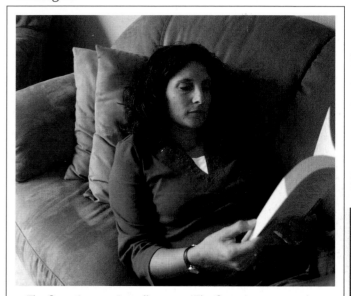

- The first trimester is really just the beginning of a lifelong journey between you and this new little life growing inside of you.

- Take time out from your busy days to reflect on how incredibly huge that is for you as a woman.

- The first trimester can be exhilarating, frightening and wonderful all at the same time.

- Well before you sense you are pregnant or feel the first kick, miraculous things are already happening!

# EMOTIONS OF PREGNANCY

## Mothers usually have a combination of emotions in early pregnancy, including joy, anxiety, and doubt

During the first thirteen weeks of pregnancy, your emotions are likely to be all over the place. One day you are excited and thrilled at the prospect of finally having a baby. The next day you are so nauseated with morning sickness that you really wonder if having a baby is worth it. Sometimes you have doubts that make you wonder if you are ready to be a mother.

Then you feel guilty for even having those thoughts when you know you should be happy about your pregnancy.

The reality is that pregnancy represents both a beginning and an end. It is the start of a new life as a mother and of learning how to take care of this precious bundle as he or she grows into adulthood. Pregnancy represents an end to

### Normal First-Trimester Emotions

- joy/excitement
- anticipation
- fear/worry
- anxiety
- doubt
- mood swings

### Up and Down

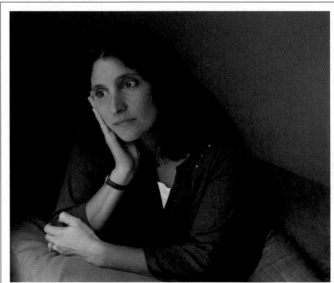

- About the only thing we can say with certainty about the emotions of early pregnancy is that it is likely for you to feel like you are on a roller coaster of emotions.

- You will be thrilled at one moment and then plummeting down from fear or worry in the next.

- Undoubtedly any number of things will be going on inside your head in the course of your day.

- Not to mention, as your physical sensations change, they can have a reciprocal effect on your roller coaster emotions as well.

spontaneity and the start of needing to make new sacrifices. You might start to think about all you have to give up during pregnancy, like having a glass of wine with dinner, or after the baby is born, needing a sitter anytime you want to go out. Not to mention that the daily responsibilities for this new life can seem incredibly daunting, especially if your own parenting role models were less than stellar.

If you have days where you feel both joy and apprehension, welcome to pregnancy! Having mixed emotions seems to go hand in hand with the first trimester of pregnancy.

····· YELLOW ● LIGHT ·············

If you happen to be one of the one in four women who are abuse survivors, experiences during pregnancy and labor can serve as painful triggers of your past hurts. The first trimester of pregnancy is an ideal time to recognize possible triggers and to learn strategies to cope. Working with a therapist, birth doula, and your care providers who are familiar with these issues will be helpful. Eventually, healing completely from the pain of abuse is possible.

## Coping

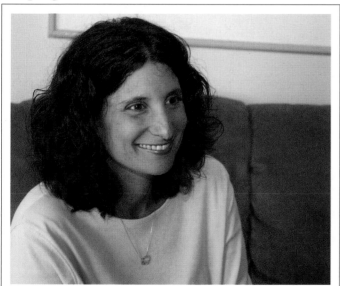

- Knowing that your topsy-turvy feelings in early pregnancy are normal and to be expected can actually be validating.

- Finding a friend or relative who hears and supports you can help you manage these emotional highs and lows.

- Friends who have had a baby themselves can provide a unique perspective to normalize your emotions.

- Some mothers also find that keeping a journal helps them to work through those emotions more constructively.

## Reflection

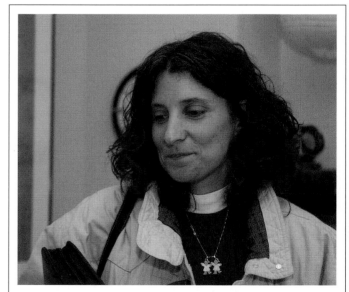

- At times it may feel like there is so much to do during pregnancy that you have no time to prepare for all of the changes happening.

- In addition to the physical changes, pregnancy is a time of great emotional, psychological, and spiritual change.

- Just like any season of your life where big changes are happening, it is important to take time for reflection.

- Add a note to your first-trimester checklist to take time out for yourself.

# PHYSICAL CHANGES

## One of the physical changes mothers may notice in the first trimester is fatigue

One of the first signs that you may notice in the first trimester is missing your period. You may also notice some breast tenderness and some irritability in your uterus that feels like your period is coming. Since the top part of your uterus, known as your fundus, presses on your bladder at this stage, you may be feeling like you have to urinate all the time.

By six weeks of pregnancy, you should get a positive result on any home pregnancy test. At around eight weeks of pregnancy, your care provider may be able to spot a bluish tinge to your cervix, known as Chadwick's sign. Another sign that is visible around six weeks is a softening of your cervical tip, called Goodell's sign. The lower segment of your uterus also

### Changes You May Notice

- missed period
- breast tenderness
- frequent urination
- fatigue
- uterine irritability
- nausea

*How Did You Know?*

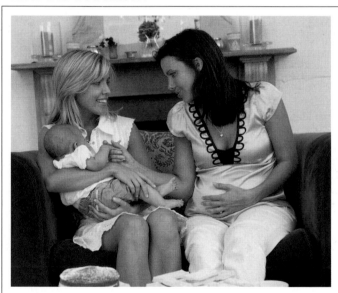

- Sometimes it can be fun to talk to other mothers about what physical sign they had that made them suspect they might be pregnant.

- You might be surprised that not all of them will say they missed their period.

- Some moms will say that they couldn't stop going to the bathroom and a friend noticed.

- Or they might have recognized that their breasts were tender well before they even missed their period.

becomes softer during the early weeks of pregnancy, and this is called Hegar's sign.

It is not at all uncommon to feel very tired in the first trimester, since the demands on your body are great. Taking care of yourself and listening to your body when you are tired are good habits to start. If you are not getting enough sleep at night, an afternoon power nap works wonders. Be sure to avoid caffeine after noon, since this can interfere with sleep.

## Changes

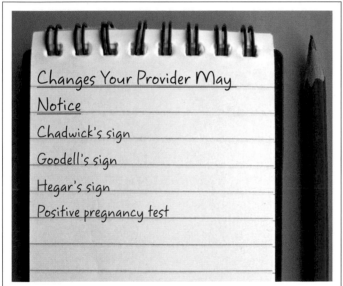

- It is a great idea to try to get an appointment with your care provider as soon as you suspect you are pregnant.

- Soon after you miss your period, you will already be several weeks into your pregnancy.

- You care provider will already be able to look at several physical changes in order to confirm your pregnancy.

- At your first appointment, be sure to talk to your care provider about any other concerns you might have about early pregnancy.

## All-day Fatigue

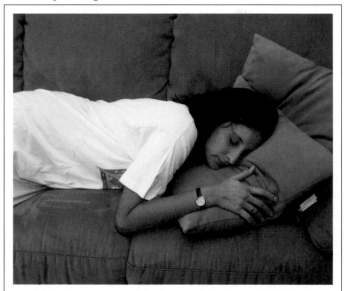

- If you are tired all day long throughout most of your first trimester, you are not alone.

- While we cannot explain the exact cause for such extreme fatigue, experts point to the rising levels of the hormone progesterone in the early weeks of pregnancy.

- Some mothers might also notice that their morning sickness symptoms contribute to their sense of fatigue.

- Be sure to listen to your body's signals by getting more rest when you need it in the early part of pregnancy.

# MANAGING MORNING SICKNESS

## The majority of expectant mothers experience some morning sickness in their first trimester

By far the most common complaint in the first trimester of pregnancy is morning sickness. About 50 to 90 percent of mothers struggle with morning sickness. Experts believe that the hormone HCG, which is secreted by the placenta in the early weeks of pregnancy, could be the main culprit behind morning sickness. Others believe that the surge of the female hormones estrogen and progesterone might be a factor in causing morning sickness. Others believe that it could result from an increase in stomach acid and a heightened sense of smell during pregnancy.

No matter the cause, morning sickness is a nuisance for many women. A few of the unluckiest mothers will develop

### Tips for Managing Morning Sickness

- Eat frequent, small, and bland meals.

- Try eating small snacks.

- Use peppermint oil (place a drop on a tissue) to sniff during waves of nausea.

- Get regular exercise.

- Try ginger in the form of tea or a lollipop.

- Eat carbohydrates such as potatoes, oatmeal, and pasta.

- Try lemons or lemonade.

- Add foods rich in vitamin B6 to your diet.

- Use acupuncture/acupressure.

- Try motion-sickness bands.

*Crackers*

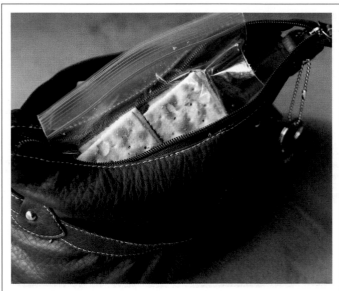

- One tried-and-true remedy for morning sickness is to eat something dry when you first get up in the morning.

- Morning sickness symptoms can be reduced during the day by keeping something in your stomach during the day.

- You will find that having an empty stomach definitely worsens symptoms of nausea.

- Saltine crackers or dry cereal are easy to keep at your bedside, throw in a snack bag and into your purse before you head out for the day.

hyperemesis gravidarum, which is severe pregnancy-related vomiting. These mothers may need to be admitted to the hospital for IV fluids to prevent or treat dehydration.

If you just found out that you are pregnant and are wondering if you are likely to have morning sickness, you will be at greater risk if you are carrying multiples, have a family history or previous pregnancy with morning sickness, suffer from migraines or motion sickness, have an overactive thyroid gland, or are thin. The good news is that there are many ways to cope with morning sickness.

## Wristbands

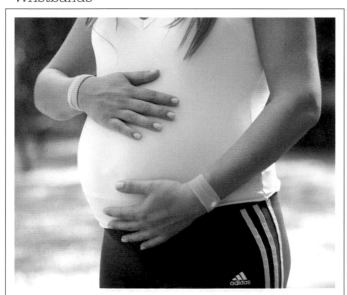

- There are several acupressure points that help to reduce nausea.

- One of those points is on the inside of your wrist, which is why mothers often find relief from wearing motion-sickness bands.

- You could also follow-up with an acupuncturist who can treat you for symptoms of nausea and vomiting.

- Since the relief from an acupuncture treatment is likely to be temporary, ask the acupuncturist to show you additional points to manage your morning sickness in between appointments.

## Lemons

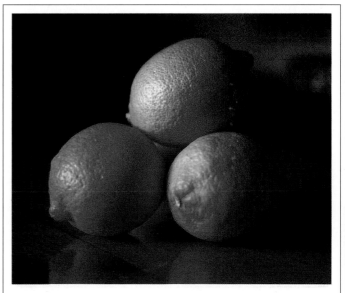

### Ginger Lemonade

2 quarts water
½ cup sugar
7 slices fresh ginger root
2 cups lemon juice (fresh squeezed)

Preparation:
Put water, sugar, and ginger root together in a saucepan and heat until boiling. Remove from heat and stir in 2 cups of fresh-squeezed lemon juice. Let it sit and cool for about 20 minutes or so, then remove the ginger root pieces. Chill your ginger lemonade before serving.

1ST TRIMESTER: MOM

# THINGS TO AVOID

## The baby's development can be affected by harmful substances such as alcohol and some medications

Most women today are aware that their growing baby can be harmed by substances in the environment as well as those they ingest, especially in the first trimester. Environmental substances include chemical fumes from paints, glues, cleaners or other potentially toxic substances. Try to reduce exposure by ventilating the appropriate areas as best you can.

Secondhand smoking also releases harmful chemicals into the air. If you work or live with someone who smokes, ask them to smoke outside to reduce your exposure.

Even if you are in the planning stages or are not sure you are pregnant yet, it is best to avoid exposure to X-rays. While there is little research about the safety of hair treatments,

Environmental Substances to Avoid

- X-rays
- salon/hair treatments
- secondary smoke
- chemical fumes

### Dental Care

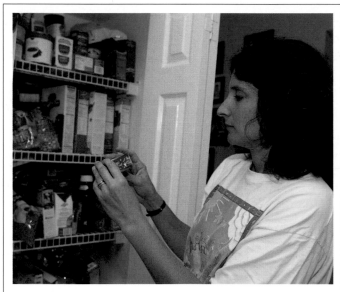

- You don't need to avoid the dentist during your pregnancy, just the X-rays, unless absolutely necessary.

- In fact, getting good dental care is crucial during pregnancy.

- Studies show that having gum disease increases your chances of preterm labor.

- So take good care of your teeth and get regular checkups for you and your baby's health.

dyes do contain chemicals. Consider avoiding hair treatments in your first trimester. Alcohol consumption during pregnancy can cause anything from subtle learning or behavioral problems to central nervous system disorders. New studies have shown that even small amounts of alcohol on a regular basis can affect your baby. Smoking increases the likelihood of miscarriage, preterm birth, and a low-birth-weight baby. Think about quitting now. If you take any prescription medications or consider using any over-the-counter drugs or herbs, first check with your care provider.

····· YELLOW ● LIGHT ·····

Some foods to consider avoiding during pregnancy include artificial sweeteners (sucralose, aspartame), non-pasteurized soft cheeses, and large fish (shark, king mackerel, swordfish, tilefish). There is not enough testing on safe limits of artificial sweeteners, soft cheeses can contain listeria, and big fish have unsafe levels of mercury.

## Ingestible Substances to Avoid

- smoking

- alcohol

- some over-the-counter medications

- some prescription medications

## Medications

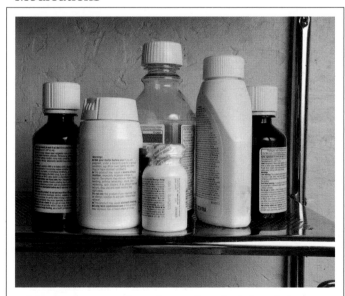

- It is easy to assume that only prescription medications need to be approved by your care provider, and to forget about safety of over-the-counter medications.

- For example, did you know that care providers do not recommend ibuprofen during pregnancy?

- Seemingly harmless over-the-counter medications can be harmful to your growing baby.

- Just to be on the safe side, check in with your care provider before you take any medication.

1ST TRIMESTER: MOM

105

# EARLY PREGNANCY & DADS
## The father can become involved in the pregnancy by finding out what is most important to mom

It is not unusual for fathers to feel a bit removed from the pregnancy at first. You may have difficulty relating to mom's changing moods and sensations. There are few visible signs of the pregnancy early on, so fathers might not have a sense of the pregnancy being real.

One thing you can do to become more involved in the pregnancy is to find out what is important to mom. What books is she reading? What are her plans for birth? You might attend prenatal visits with her. This gives you the opportunity to ask questions about issues such as prenatal testing and childbirth.

A common emotional reaction to pregnancy is that fathers have a deepening sense of their role as provider. They may

### Tips on Getting Involved

- Ask mom what she needs.
- Find out what is important to her.
- Attend prenatal visits.
- Read pregnancy books.
- Take care of mom.

*Dads at Work*

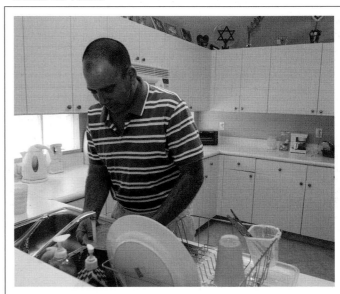

- Although fathers may find that some support comes from their friendships at work, be cautious of the advice from well-meaning co-workers.

- It is all too common to hear all the horror stories of labor, not to mention other fathers who can't resist telling you what to do.

- Remember your role is to support your wife in what is important to her.

- Your relationship will only be enhanced when you work together in making important decisions.

take a hard look at finances and seek a higher-paying job or a second job in order to meet the demands of a growing family.

This is also a time when dads might start thinking about their ability to be a father. What is/was your relationship with your father like? Talking to your friends who are already fathers can be a help right now. When your own fatherhood is on the horizon, it is helpful to re-examine your parenting role models so that you learn to be the best father possible for your baby.

## Reading and Sharing Opinions

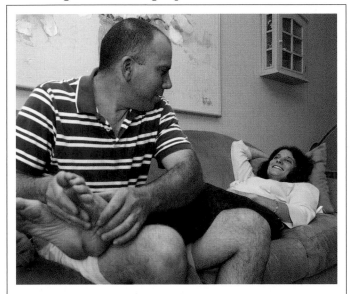

- Some fathers are interested in reading every book that mom has read.

- Others are not as enthusiastic about reading but might prefer watching DVDs or taking classes.

- Even if you only have time to read a few pages in each chapter of your pregnancy books, you will feel much more confident in your role if you are informed.

- Your opinion matters, too; research your options right alongside of mom so that you can be fully invested in those decisions. Share your opinions with one another.

## Helping Out

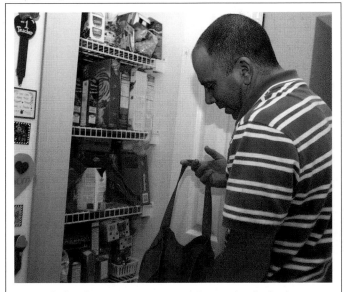

- As a dad-to-be, you are not the one who is responsible for eating well and resting.

- Think about how you can use your own gifts and talents to help her during pregnancy.

- You can lend a few extra hours a week to help with housework. Your help will ensure she is getting the additional rest she needs in the first trimester.

- If you are a planner, you can help her with research and looking ahead to the next stage.

# BABY'S NUTRITIONAL NEEDS

## The nutrients mother eats can affect the long-term health of her baby as an adult

Now there is even greater motivation to choose a salad for lunch instead of french fries. Research shows that your baby's long-term health can be affected by what you eat during pregnancy.

Dr. Peter Nathanielsz has discovered that when there is a lack of adequate nutrients in the mother's diet, the baby's organs are forced to compensate. The baby's body sends available nutrients to the most vital organs, such as the brain and heart, and away from other developing organs.

Dr. Nathanielsz explains that this is observed in how the baby's liver grows. If nutrients are limited, the baby's body has to send nutrient supply to the heart and brain and away from

*Mother's Diet Affects Baby's:*

- weight as an adult.

- blood pressure later in life.

- blood sugar profile in adulthood.

- lifelong cardiovascular health.

### Prenatal Vitamins

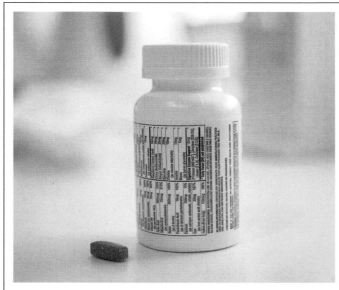

- Let's face it: Certain days you are not going to eat as well as you should during your pregnancy.

- Taking prenatal vitamins every day is a good "insurance policy" so that you and your baby are getting the crucial vitamins and minerals you will need.

- If your stomach is bothered by prenatal vitamins, take them at night.

- You could also try a different brand or see if a liquid or chewable form is a bit easier on your stomach.

organs such as the liver. The liver grows smaller than normal. A small liver that cannot adequately control cholesterol may lead to high cholesterol later in your baby's adult life.

Based on Dr. Nathanielsz' research, a lack of nutrients during pregnancy can also lead to type 2 diabetes, obesity, hypertension, and heart disease. There is reason to believe that if your daughter's health is affected, so may be the health of her children. The good news is that eating healthy foods and taking prenatal vitamins is healthy for both your children and your grandchildren!

## Adding Nutrients

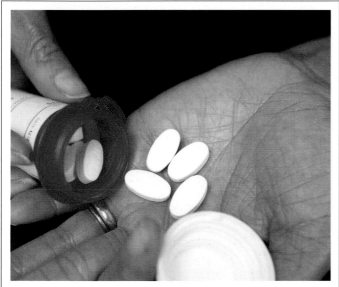

- You can easily find ways to add more nutrients to your diet.

- In addition to fresh produce, you can also buy frozen fruits and vegetables when they are not available in season.

- Add fruit to your breakfast cereal, nuts to your salad, and lettuce and tomatoes to your sandwich.

- Throw extra vegetables in your slow-cooker meal for dinner for added vitamins.

## Nutrition

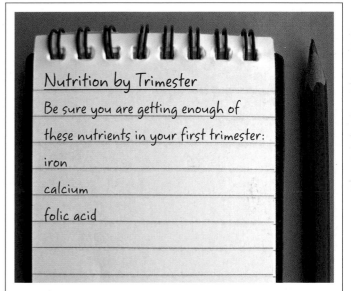

- A variety of nutrients are important for a healthy pregnancy.

- Highlighted here are several that play a vital role in the first trimester.

- Folic acid is needed to prevent neural tube defects. Calcium is important for your baby's developing bones and iron is needed for blood stores.

- Be sure that your first trimester diet is packed with these and other nutrients to be sure you and your baby are getting what you need.

1ST TRIMESTER: BABY

# STAYING RELAXED

## Mothers and their growing babies can benefit from taking time out for relaxation

It seems that all of us suffer from varying amounts of stress at different times in our lives. Pregnancy can add additional stress to daily life in many ways. Coping with all of the changes in your body can be stressful to some mothers. Making decisions about prenatal tests and what to do with test results is nearly always stressful. Both mothers and fathers can have

stress about the financial burden of raising children, especially given the rising costs of college tuition! Stress is not good for us. Not only does stress negatively affect moms during pregnancy, it can also lead to more allergies and asthma in babies, according to a study done by Dr. Rosalind Wright, which was funded by the U.S. National Heart, Lung, and Blood Institute.

### Relaxation Exercise: Part 1

- Get into a comfortable position.

- Start by taking your stressful thoughts from your day and putting them aside.

- Allow your body and mind to relax now.

- Close your eyes and take some slow, deep breaths.

- First focus on your forehead and face muscles.

- Take a deep breath, and as you exhale, think about relaxing those muscles.

- Think about your neck and shoulders. Are they tense?

- As you breathe deeply, let your shoulders fall and your neck muscles soften.

*Relaxation Exercises: Part 2*

- Each arm should be soft, loose, and heavy. Take a deep breath; breathe away any tension in your arms.

- Check your hands. Are they open and not clenched? Are your fingers relaxed? Take another deep breath.

- Now focus on your back.

- Wherever you feel tension, breathe it away.

- Your hips and pelvis should be loose and heavy. Breathe again to relax them. Now picture the muscles in your buttocks.

- Take a deep breath and relax those muscles.

Here are some simple things you can do to give you a better sense of control in your life—to reduce stress when it feels like you have lost control! Learn to prioritize. Not everything is urgent, so let things wait that can wait. Remember to say no sometimes. A lot of stress comes from over-committing yourself. Take a break from the stress. Go outside, or go away for the weekend.

You might think about talking to a friend who is a good listener. Be sure you are getting adequate sleep and eating healthily. Find out what helps you relax better. You might enjoy a bath, massage, or a relaxation exercise as often as possible. Some folks find that prayer or meditation is stress-relieving. If you are still struggling with stress, seek a counselor for help.

## Relaxation Exercises: Part 3

- As you focus on your thighs, they should be relaxed.

- Breathe now and relax them.

- Now relax your calves.

- Focus on your ankles, feet, and toes. Breathe to relax them.

- Now as you think about your entire body, is it soft? Find the tension wherever it may be.

- Take several deep breaths and let your entire body enjoy that relaxation.

- There is no hurry to get up.

- Stay here for several minutes, enjoying the relaxation of your entire body.

- When you are ready, you may open your eyes and get up.

### Benefits of Relaxation

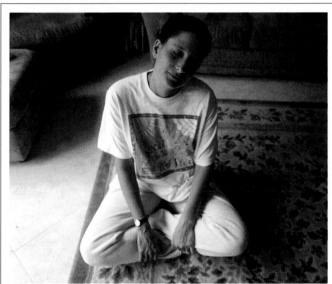

- Relaxation lowers your blood pressure and heart rate.

- It also reduces your levels of stress hormones.

- Relaxation increases the blood flow to your vital organs, including your uterus.

- You may find that symptoms such as headaches and fatigue are reduced by relaxation.

# SHARING YOUR BIG NEWS

## Waiting until the heartbeat is detectable may be a good time for parents to share their big news

Do you call your parents as soon as your pregnancy is confirmed, or do you wait until after the first trimester is over? This can be a dilemma for some expectant parents. What is right for one family may not be what is right for another.

Pregnancy is exciting for everyone, so having to wait three months before sharing your news may be nearly impossible!

You may want your friends and family to be included in the pregnancy as soon as possible.

The argument against sharing your news in the first trimester is that there is a higher chance of miscarriage during this time. Some parents might feel that they want to protect their family from knowing or asking questions about the

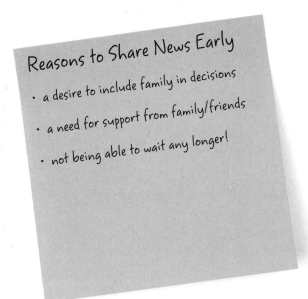

Reasons to Share News Early

• a desire to include family in decisions

• a need for support from family/friends

• not being able to wait any longer!

*Deciding to Wait*

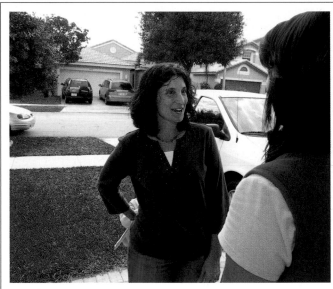

- It is not unusual to hear that mothers would rather wait longer to share their news.

- You may prefer to wait if you have had complications with your pregnancies and you want to be sure everything is going well.

- If you feel that your family may not be supportive of your pregnancy, some mothers choose to wait until they are ready.

- A good rule of thumb is to share your news when you are ready and to your closest circle of friends and family.

pregnancy if things don't turn out as they had hoped. If you have had a history of one or more miscarriages, it would be understandable that you would want to wait longer before sharing the news about your current pregnancy.

Perhaps a good compromise would be to wait until after your baby's heartbeat has been detected, around eight weeks. By then your risk of miscarriage is only 1.5 percent. You may also choose to wait until after your first trimester is nearly over to share your big news.

•••••••••••••••• RED ● LIGHT ••••••••••••
How do you identify a miscarriage? A miscarriage prior to six weeks of pregnancy results in bleeding that looks like a heavy period. A miscarriage between six and twelve weeks of pregnancy results in moderate pain/cramping in addition to bleeding. A miscarriage more than twelve weeks into pregnancy results in bleeding and pain that feels similar to labor. If you have any bleeding in pregnancy, contact your care provider.

## Privacy Differences

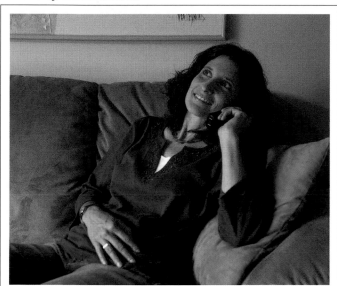

- Some expectant parents share every detail with their families.

- Others have a different level of privacy with each other.

- Many agree it is best to share early news only with close friends and fam-ily, leaving out distant acquaintances.

- Chances are high that each expectant couple will know when and how to share this news as well as other details of the pregnancy with their own families.

## Creative Ways to Share

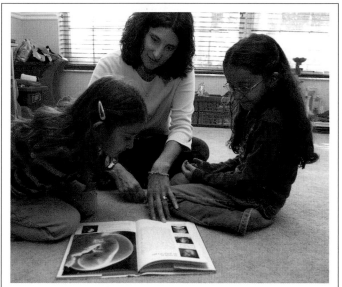

- There are plenty of creative ways to share your big news with friends and family.

- Some mothers frame a copy of their ultrasound image and give it to their parents as a gift.

- You could find a T-shirt or sweatshirt with a message for the new grandparents, such as "Best Grandparents," and give it to them at the next holiday.

- Or wrap up a child's toy or book and enclose a note to the grandparents that says something like "please read/play this with me in six months!"

# THE FIRST MONTH

## In the first month your baby starts with two cells and by four weeks has a beating heart

Even before you may start to recognize the earliest signs of pregnancy, your baby begins to make amazing changes. Ovulation and conception occur approximately two weeks after the first day of your last menstrual period. The tiny sperm travel up through the uterus into your fallopian tube, and one will penetrate the lining of the egg released by your ovary. The process of the sperm meeting the egg can take as little as five minutes or as long as a few days.

The two-celled structure now begins to rapidly divide into a bundle of cells. By week three, the tiny embryo makes its three-to-four-day journey down the fallopian tube to the uterus. A small cavity separates the embryo into two sections;

### Highlights at One Month

- conception
- cells divide
- embryo implants
- placenta attaches
- germ layers form

*Preparation and Conception*

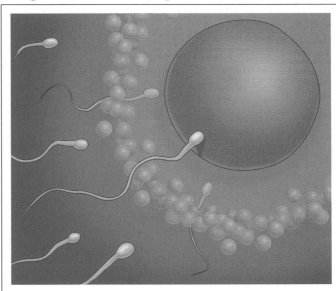

- Right after you ovulate, the ruptured ovarian follicle turns into the corpus luteum.

- The corpus luteum secretes progesterone and estrogen to prepare the uterine lining.

- After ovulation the egg meets the sperm in the fallopian tube, and conception occurs.

- The fertilized egg remains in the fallopian tube for three to four days.

one becomes your growing baby (called the embryoblast) and the other becomes the placenta (called the trophoblast). By the seventeenth day after conception, the trophoblast secretes an enzyme that helps the little embryo attach itself to the lining of your uterus. During the third week, germ layers begin to form that become the baby's skin, nervous system, internal organs, and skeletal system. By the end of the third week, your baby will already have a beating heart that is circulating blood throughout its tiny body, which at that point is only $1/_5$ centimeter long.

## Cell Division and Implantation

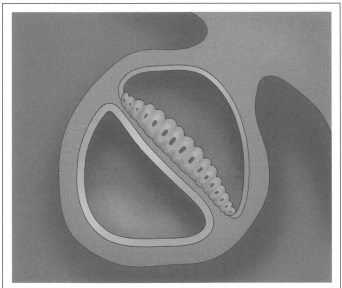

- Within twenty-four hours of fertilization, the two cells have begun to rapidly divide.

- The tiny solid bundle of cells soon becomes a hollow ball of cells called a blastocyst.

- Right before implantation the blastocyst breaks out of its covering.

- As it meets the uterine lining, hormones are exchanged and the blastocyst attaches.

## Embryo Is Here

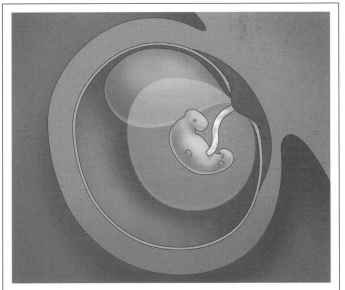

- By three weeks the little bundle of cells is now called an embryo.

- Major developments are occurring in your baby's digestive, nervous, and skeletal systems.

- The little embryo is only about the size of a pea.

- Do you know you are pregnant?

# THE SECOND MONTH

## All of your baby's major organs are formed by the second month of pregnancy

The second month of pregnancy is a very exciting time in your baby's growth. As you move into week five, your baby's brain begins to divide into three sections: the hindbrain, midbrain, and forebrain. Your baby's forebrain starts to grow into your baby's nose and eyes. Believe it or not, your baby's heart is already busy growing into a four-chambered organ. By week six of pregnancy, the skeletal system, including bones in your baby's shoulders, arms, hips, and legs, makes its first appearance. Even your baby's blood type is already established by six weeks.

At the end of the seventh week, we have hit a huge landmark in your baby's development. Every major organ system

### Highlights at Two Months

- brain divides into three sections
- heart develops into four chambers
- bones grow in shoulders, arms, and legs
- blood type present
- liver makes red blood cells
- heartbeat detected on ultrasound

### Baby's Development

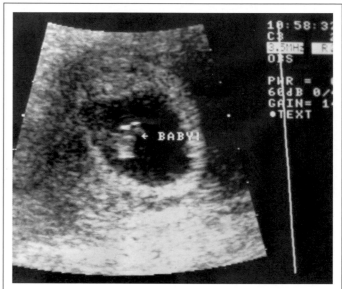

- Even though there are no joints yet, the bones in your baby's arms and legs are starting to form at the beginning of the second month.

- These little limbs will gradually lengthen and eventually begin moving in just a few weeks.

- By the end of your second month, your baby will already have definitive muscles in his/her head, limbs and trunk.

- Believe it or not, your baby actually has a tail in the first few weeks of pregnancy, which nearly disappears by the end of the eighth week.

is now present in its earliest form! Did you know that your baby's liver is already beginning to make red blood cells and that your baby's arms and legs can move spontaneously? Your baby's heartbeat could be detected on an ultrasound by week six of pregnancy. Hormones produced this week will start to form your baby's reproductive organs. Even nerve fibers have started to travel across your baby's body and the earliest brain waves have been detected. What an amazing journey we can already see unfolding in this little embryo.

## Major Organs

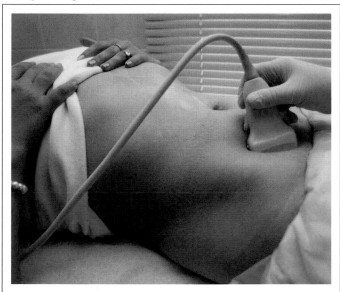

- By the end of week seven, your baby's major organs are all present.

- This is one of the most sensitive periods in your pregnancy.

- For this reason, it is important to avoid any exposure to harmful substances.

- You may be just starting to realize that you are pregnant, since you have now missed a period by several weeks.

## Nervous System

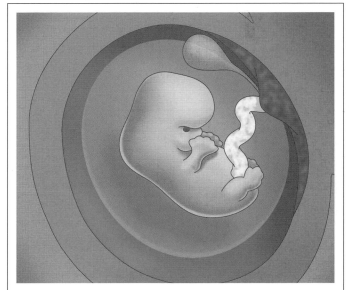

- You might not imagine that your baby's brain is developing this soon, but it is.

- Your baby's cerebral cortex, which is the area that plays a role in memories, thought, and language, is beginning to grow cells.

- Even cerebrospinal fluid is already present and beginning to circulate.

- Your baby's spinal cord grows all the way down the entire length of the spine by the end of the second month.

1ST TRIMESTER: BABY

# THE THIRD MONTH

## The embryo becomes a fetus and will have functioning kidneys by the end of this month

As you move into your third month of pregnancy, your baby's development continues at a rapid pace. The beginning of the fetal stage occurs at nine weeks and lasts through the end of your pregnancy. Believe it or not, differences between males and females can be distinguished now. Your baby's kidneys make such huge changes that by nine weeks they begin

to function, and by twelve weeks they will already begin to secrete urine.

Another interesting development is that your baby's adrenal glands begin to produce a hormone, called cortisol, which helps him or her with the stress response. The spinal cord has grown all the way to the end of your baby's body.

### Highlights at Three Months

- embryo becomes a fetus
- kidneys begin to function
- adrenals produce cortisol
- fingernails/toenails appear
- heartbeat is detected in Doppler
- taste buds appear
- vocal cords appear

*Size of Your Baby*

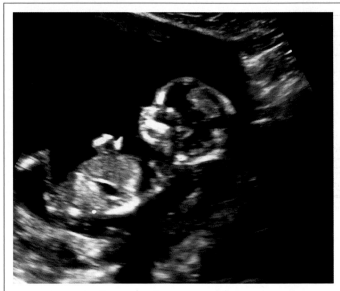

- Your baby is still very small at three months, but his/her little body is developing rapidly.

- Your baby is about 3 to 5 centimeters long by ten weeks of pregnancy.

- To put that into perspective, that is a little less than 2 inches in length.

- Her weight is about four grams, which is approximately the same weight as four dimes.

Fingernails and toenails appear at the very tips of your baby's toes and fingers during week ten.

Your care provider may be able to detect your baby's breathing movements in an ultrasound as early as week eleven, although it is more likely that these movements won't be seen for a few more weeks. At week twelve your baby's lungs already have their oval shape. Even your baby's taste buds and vocal cords have appeared. All of these amazing changes in the first trimester are the main reason why it is so important to take such good care of you.

## Baby's Appearance

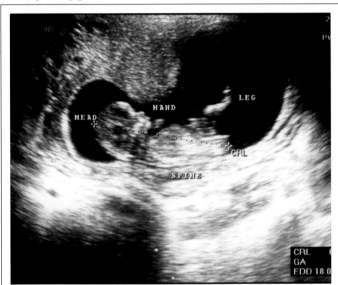

- Can you imagine that as small as your baby is, the tiniest tips of her fingernails and toenails have already appeared at the ends of her fingers and toes?

- Your baby starts to look much more human-like this month with the head more rounded and her skin now pink in color.

- However your baby's head is still proportionately large compared to the body.

- Even the very early beginnings of your baby's external sex organs are visible by the end of the week twelve.

## Baby Is a Fetus!

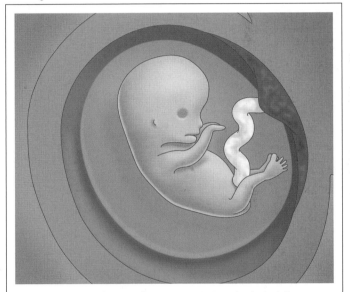

- Starting at week nine of pregnancy and continuing all the way to the end of gestation, your baby is now considered a fetus.

- By week eleven of pregnancy, your care provider would be able to hear your baby's heartbeat with a Dopplar at your prenatal visit.

- Having the baby's heartbeat confirmed is one of the most exciting things that women report about being pregnant!

- Congratulations on completing your first trimester with success!

# YOUR SECOND-TRIMESTER CHECKLIST

## Mothers will need to add 300 more calories to their daily total starting in their second trimester

The second trimester is the first time you will need to increase your intake of calories. During both the second and third trimesters, you should add an additional 300 calories to your daily intake. This might seem like a lot, but it is only the equivalent of about 2 tablespoons of granola and a container of yogurt, or two average-size slices of bread.

One of the biggest concerns women have is how much weight they should gain and how much is too much. The newest recommendations for your pregnancy weight gain are based on your body mass index (BMI) before you became pregnant. From there you can determine how much weight you should be gaining throughout your pregnancy.

*Second-Trimester Checklist*

- Add 300 calories per day.

- Interview and select a pediatrician.

- Make decisions about work/day care.

- Register for childbirth classes.

- Continue your healthy diet.

- Continue reading.

*Formula for BMI*

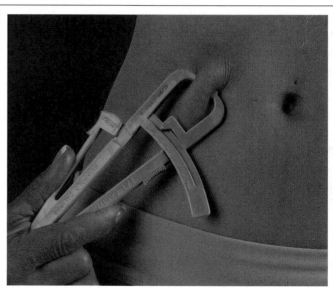

- Weight (pounds) / Height (inches) / Height (inches) multiplied by 703

Example:

- 130-pound woman, 5 feet 6 inches tall

- Take 130 and divide by 66 inches = 1.96.

- Divide 1.96 by 66 again = .029.

- Multiply .029 by 703.

- BMI is 20.98.

Once you have figured out your BMI, you can review the chart below to see what weight category you fall into and how much weight you should gain during pregnancy. For example, a woman who is at her ideal weight should gain between 26 and 32 pounds.

Unless you have already done so, your second trimester should include making decisions about returning to work, day-care options, and finding a pediatrician and registering for childbirth classes.

**ZOOM**

Did you know that one reason your body makes added fat stores during pregnancy is to prepare you for breastfeeding? If you breastfeed your baby, your body uses up twenty-four calories per ounce, or about 500 or more calories every day.

**Chart – BMI and Weight Gain**

| Category | BMI | Recommended Weight Gain |
|---|---|---|
| Underweight | Under 19.8 | 27.5–40 pounds |
| Normal Weight | 19.8–26.0 | 25–32 pounds |
| Overweight | 26.0–29 | 15–25 pounds |
| Obese | Over 29 | 15 pounds |

**Where Does All Your Pregnancy Weight Go?**

- Baby: 7½ pounds
- Placenta: 1 pound
- Uterus: 2 pounds
- Amniotic fluid: 2 pounds
- Breasts: 1 pound
- Blood volume: 2½ pounds
- Fat: 5 pounds
- Tissue fluid: 6 pounds
- Total: 27 pounds

# EMOTIONS OF SECOND TRIMESTER

## The decision to return to work or stay home can be an emotional one for many mothers

One of the definite changes in the second trimester of pregnancy is that sensations are becoming more familiar. You might be feeling more confident in managing the changes in pregnancy as well as learning the routines of eating well and taking care of yourself. You usually have renewed energy and are sleeping well in your second trimester.

Though some mothers make decisions about returning to work or staying home even before they become pregnant, exploring your work options should take place no later than your second trimester. We feel it is important to discuss this within the framework of pregnancy emotions because work-related decisions for new moms can be laden with emotions.

### Home-based Day Care

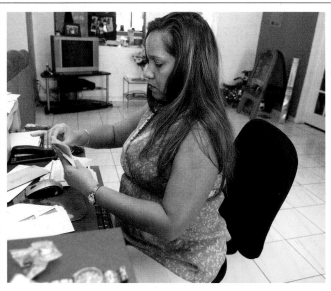

- One of the most popular options for working parents is to find a day-care provider who takes care of children in his or her home.

- Look for someone who is licensed by the state in which you live.

- Ask if the in-home day-care provider is certified in CPR and has a background check to show you.

- Find out what the backup plan is for illness or emergencies with the provider.

### Day-care Center

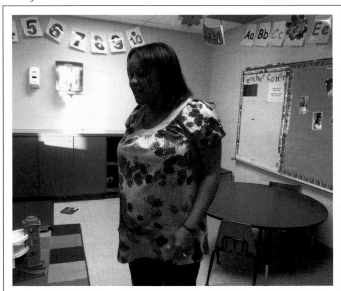

- Parents may enjoy the structure of a day-care center environment for their children.

- Be sure to ask if the day-care center is accredited and if background checks are done for all staff.

- If you will not be working full-time, do they offer flex hours or part-time day care?

- Ask about any holiday schedules, availability, and ratios of adults to children.

A growing number of women have home-based businesses. Another popular option is to work part-time away from home and be at home for the rest of the week. If you plan to return to work full-time, various child-care options include using a day-care center, a home-based child-care provider, hiring a private, or shared, nanny or using family.

Making this decision for your family is not an easy one. Evaluate your own needs and goals, talk to your partner, and consider what works best for you.

## MAKE IT EASY

The average cost for one child in full-time day care is $8,000 per year with a low of $4,000 and a high of $14,000 in some areas. Start with your salary, subtract day-care costs, costs for clothing, gas, and any other work-related expenses, and see what is left over. When baby number two arrives, the cost of day care will be much more challenging for parents.

### Nanny or Au Pair

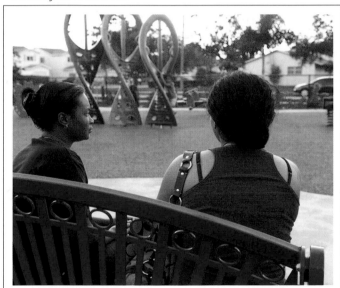

- Some families hire a private nanny or au pair, or share them with another family.

- Both of these providers should also come with CPR certification and background checks.

- Costs for a nanny per week can run between $350 and $700.

- Au pairs get a weekly stipend closer to $200; however, the host family also provides lodging, food, education fees, car insurance, and airfare as well as initial program fees.

### Benefits of Staying at Home

- saves money
- sense of satisfaction
- spend more time with children
- more relaxed schedule
- makes home schooling possible

# PHYSICAL CHANGES

## Mothers may notice their very first Braxton-Hicks contractions during their second trimester

Moms are thrilled to discover that frequently their morning sickness ebbs in their second trimester. Because of the increased circulation in your pelvic floor, you might be feeling more romantic during this time. You might think about planning a weekend getaway now.

Some of the other changes you may notice in your second trimester are multiple changes in your skin. You may notice that your pigment is darker around your nipple tissue. Some mothers notice pigment changes in their face and even a dark line that appears straight down the middle of their abdomen, known as the linea nigra. Stretch marks in your lower abdomen, hips, thighs, and breasts can also start at the

### Changes You May Notice

- increased desire for sex
- more energy
- skin changes
- Braxton-Hicks contractions
- stretch marks
- colostrum

### Braxton-Hicks Contractions

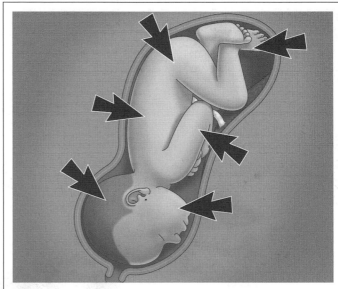

- Braxton-Hicks contractions are named after the physician who identified these "practice" contractions of your uterus.

- They usually feel like a tightening in your belly for a minute or two, then a release. They may last for many minutes, especially if you are very active.

- They do not strengthen in intensity or get closer together.

- Call your care provider if you notice more than six contractions per hour that do not go away with rest and fluids.

end of the second trimester. Other breast changes include the appearance of colostrum, which looks like a pale yellow discharge that you might see in your bra. Colostrum is the first milk your breasts produce before true breast milk comes between two and five days after birth. Your very first Braxton-Hicks contractions might also begin in your second trimester. Braxton-Hicks contractions will feel like a tightening around your belly, feeling like your baby is curling up into a tight ball. These are easy to distinguish from labor contractions in that they do not increase in intensity or frequency.

**ZOOM**

Great product marketing has led many pregnant women to believe that certain skin-care creams can prevent stretch marks from appearing. The truth is that research does not show that any skin-care cream, including those with cocoa butter, prevents stretch marks.

## Stretch Marks

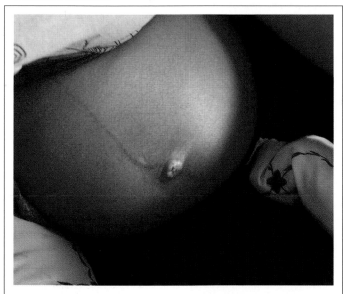

- Some mothers will notice stretch marks starting in their second trimester or as late as their third trimester.

- You are more likely to get stretch marks if you have a family history, you are over-weight, or you are carrying a large baby or multiples.

- Hydrating well and elimi-nating empty calories may help reduce stretch marks.

- To try to reduce stretch marks, use products that contain ingredients to replenish your skin such as vitamin E and aloe vera.

## Intimacy

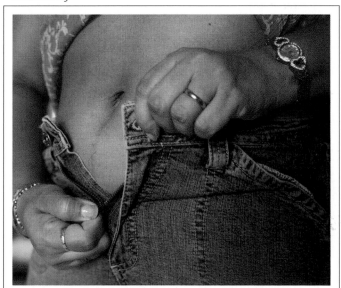

- Many mothers report that the second trimester makes them feel a desire for inti-macy and sex.

- Now that your morning sickness has receded, the second trimester is the best window to rekindle romance.

- Most couples can enjoy a normal sex life during pregnancy.

- However, if you have any concerns about whether or not it is safe for you to make love during preg-nancy, check with your care provider.

# MANAGING COMPLICATIONS

## How to read symptoms and get help during pregnancy challenges is important in the second trimester

Although most mothers find that their pregnancy proceeds without a hitch, a few moms hit some bumps in the road. One of those bumps can be finding out that you have gestational diabetes. About 3 to 10 percent of mothers will develop gestational diabetes during pregnancy.

Toward the end of the second trimester, your care provider will recommend that you take an oral glucose challenge screening test. If your results are positive on the screening test, you will be asked to take a three-hour glucose tolerance diagnostic test (OGTT). A positive result on the OGTT requires that you follow a diabetic diet that restricts simple sugars, getting regular exercise, and routinely checking your blood sugar at

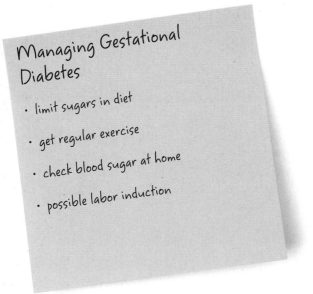

Managing Gestational Diabetes

- limit sugars in diet
- get regular exercise
- check blood sugar at home
- possible labor induction

*Blood Glucose Testing*

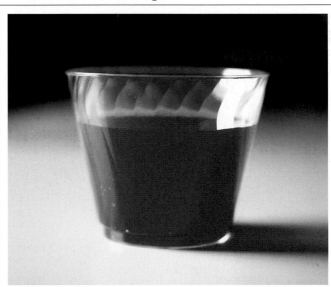

- Your provider may recommend that your blood sugar be checked one hour after each meal.

- You are twice as likely to develop high blood pressure if you have gestational diabetes, so your provider will monitor your BP frequently.

- If you are not able to manage your blood sugar levels after two weeks of diet and exercise, your provider may recommend oral medications or regular insulin injections.

home. You might also need to take medicine to control your sugar levels if you can't control them with dietary changes.

Another bump that can happen during pregnancy is that your blood pressure can become elevated. This is known as pregnancy-induced hypertension (PIH). It is more likely for you to have PIH if you already have a history of hypertension in your family or if this is your first baby. Your provider will be monitoring your blood pressure and testing for the presence of protein in your urine. You may be asked to limit your activity, lie on your left side, and increase your fluid intake.

## RED LIGHT

Signs of preterm labor to watch for between twenty and thirty-seven weeks of pregnancy: pelvic pressure (feels like the baby is pressing down in your abdomen or rectum); low, dull back pain; cramping (similar to menstrual cramps); uterine contractions that occur ten minutes or closer together with or without discomfort; or intestinal cramping with or without diarrhea. Call your care provider as soon as you notice any of the above symptoms.

### Blood Pressure

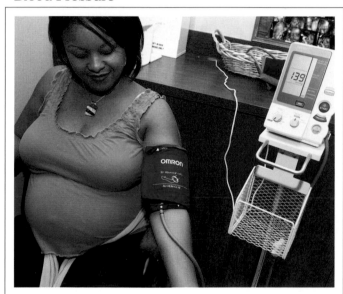

- You may have wondered why your blood pressure and urine is checked at every prenatal visit.

- If your BP becomes elevated beyond a normal range but returns to normal when you lie down, you may be advised to cut back on your activities and rest more.

- Your care provider will also be checking your urine sample for protein at your visits.

- This is one way to diagnose if your PIH is developing into preeclampsia.

### Bed Rest

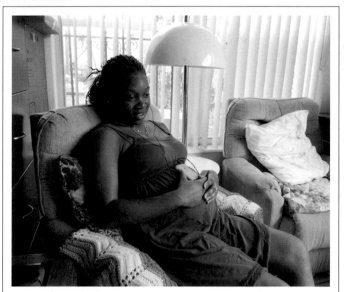

- Bed rest is commonly prescribed for both preterm labor and pregnancy-induced hypertension.

- Resting on your side is also the best position for circulation and blood return from your extremities to your heart.

- However, bed rest can be a challenge for women who are active during pregnancy.

- Thankfully most moms have laptops and cell phones to save them from complete boredom.

# CHOOSING A PEDIATRICIAN

## Parents should look for separate areas for sick and well children in the pediatrician's office

Interviewing a pediatrician should also be on your second-trimester checklist. He or she will need to be a trusted professional that you can call on for advice. You should feel comfortable with his or her recommendations.

First impressions count when you make your first contact with a prospective pediatrician. Are you put on hold for a

long time? Is the staff responsive to your needs?

When you walk in, get an overview of your surroundings. Notice if the reception area is clean and inviting. Is there enough seating for both adults and children? If the reception area is crammed with people, you might wonder how busy the practice is. Is the waiting room separated into areas for

### Things to Notice

- How is your phone call handled?

- How are you treated by the staff?

- Is reception area roomy, clean, and inviting?

- Are there separate well-child and sick-child areas?

- Are exam rooms clean?

*Responsiveness and Availability*

- As you schedule an interview, imagine calling with a sick baby at home.

- A ten-minute wait to talk to a receptionist will not feel stressful to you now, but it will if you are worried about your baby.

- What is the doctor's availability to meet with you?

- Based on the response you get, you may know how quickly your needs will be attended to when your baby is a patient.

sick versus healthy children? Once you meet the pediatrician, ask if she has appointments first thing in the morning just for newborns, which is sometimes offered to avoid exposure to sick children. Check if this pediatrician has privileges at your place of birth and whether routine visits can be scheduled with one particular doctor. Parents who have strong preferences about immunizations will want to be sure that their pediatrician shares that philosophy.

## MAKE IT EASY

Is Your Pediatrician Breastfeeding-Friendly? Is your pediatrician recommended by La Leche League or lactation consultants? What recommendations would they make for breastfeeding problems? Has the staff had breastfeeding training? How long would they recommend breastfeeding? What breastfeeding sources does he/she recommend? Can you breastfeed during procedures?

## Environment

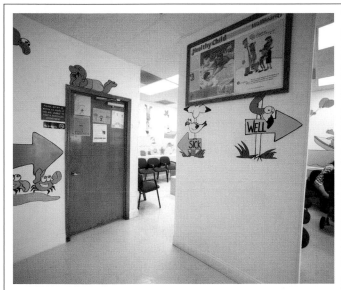

- Any experienced mother will tell you that the pediatrician's office is always crawling with viruses and bacteria.

- The last thing you will want is for your healthy baby to get sick after a routine checkup at your pediatrician's office.

- Be sure there are separate rooms for sick and well children and that the toys do not gravitate from room to room.

- Holding your baby close to you in a sling rather than in a stroller or infant seat will also help to reduce exposure when you are out.

### Questions to Ask

- Do you have early morning appointments for newborns?

- Can I see you consistently or will we be rotated among the doctors?

- Do you have privileges at my place of birth?

- What is your philosophy regarding immunizations?

- How can we get in touch with you after hours?

# DAD'S ROLE

## Dads can help mothers shop for necessary baby items during the second trimester

So much of pregnancy is centered on the health and well-being of the baby and mother that dads can be forgotten. You do have a role and a very important one at that! Now is a perfect time to start getting even more involved in your wife's pregnancy if you have not already done so. Here are some ideas to help you feel more like a part of this exciting event.

Grab a few of the best pregnancy, birth, or parenting books and read a bit before you go to bed. If you have trouble reading several books in their entirety, ask if mom can highlight the most important parts of each book that she wants to share with you. Remember that the more you read, the more helpful you can be during pregnancy in selecting care

### Tips on Getting Involved

- Read up on pregnancy, birth, and post-partum adjustment.
- Help interview the pediatrician.
- Help select a childbirth class.
- Review baby needs.
- Shop for baby items.
- Read to your baby.

*Making Decisions*

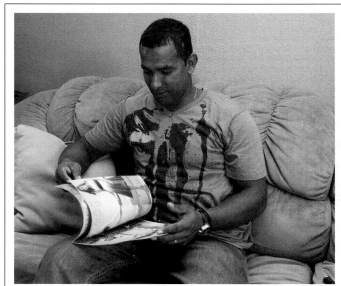

- Dads can attend prenatal visits and help interview care providers and doulas during pregnancy.
- Other ways that fathers can be supportive is with decisions about day-care options.
- Remember that the more you and your wife work together and make decisions as a team, the healthier your marriage will be.
- Remember that supporting one another and managing challenges is something you will do together for the rest of your lives.

providers and classes, helping in the birth plan, and assisting your partner as she goes through birth.

You also might enjoy helping mom identify what she needs and then shopping for some of the baby items during pregnancy. The second trimester is an ideal time to see what items you might be able to borrow, put on the shower gift registry, or purchase in advance. If you enjoy shopping online, perhaps you can find gently used items on eBay as a way of getting involved.

## MAKE IT EASY

Did you know that from twenty-four weeks of pregnancy, your baby's sense of hearing is completely developed? This gives you a wonderful opportunity to read or talk to your growing baby so that your voice is familiar to him or her after birth.

### Shopping

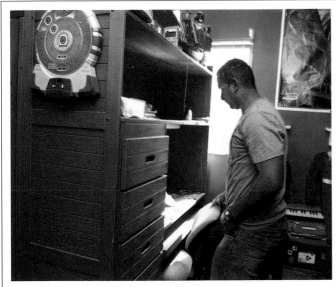

- Mom may not ask you to go shopping to pick out baby things with her, but offer to tag along.

- You might enjoy helping her pick out some new things for the baby.

- Besides, her excitement over picturing your baby in cute outfits will be quite contagious.

- Not to mention your muscles will come in handy when all of the baby items need to be loaded into the car.

### Online Bargains

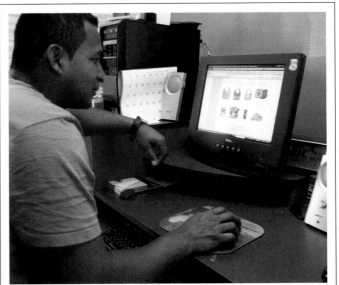

- Dads are often very interested in the various ways they can save money.

- Online shopping is one of the best ways to save on time and gas.

- Many internet sites allow you to do price comparisons among various companies to get the lowest prices.

- This can be a huge relief for Mom and one contribution you can make to show her that you care.

# THE BABY NURSERY

## Crib safety is one of the most important aspects of planning your baby nursery

Now is the best time to decide what furniture or equipment you will need in the nursery. Some of the functional items include a crib, changing table, bassinet, rocker or glider, and a dresser. Bassinets can be used for napping during the day in the main part of the house or for the parents' room. However, most babies will outgrow a bassinet after three months,

so eventually you will need to purchase a crib. If you acquire a previously owned crib, be sure to check it for crib safety guidelines.

Check that the end panels are solid and not decorative and that the corner posts are flush with the rest of the panels. If it's an older crib that has been passed down, make sure there

## Tips on Crib Safety

- solid, not decorative end panels

- distance between slats no more than $2^3/_8$ inches apart

- corner posts flush with other panels

- mattress same size as crib, with no gaps

- no blankets, pillows, or soft toys in crib

### More about Cribs

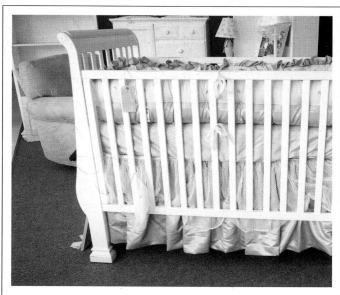

- Sometimes changing your baby right in the crib can be convenient.

- This is another way to cut some costs if you cannot afford a separate changing table.

- Be sure the lowered crib sides are at least 9 inches above the mattress to prevent the baby from accidentally falling out.

- Look for a locking, hand-operated latch for the dropped sides that will not release unintentionally.

is no peeling paint. Also, check the mattress size to make sure it is the same size as the crib, with no gaps. If you can fit two fingers side by side between the mattress and the side of the crib, do not use the crib. Stuffed animals make popular shower gifts, but do not place them in the baby's crib. In addition, your baby's crib should be free of blankets, pillows, or any other items, all of which may be smothering hazards to the baby.

Having comfortable seating for late-night feedings is helpful in your nursery. Gliders are a popular baby nursery purchase, but before you purchase one, sit in it with a breastfeeding pillow on your lap so you can see if you have enough room on either side for your baby. Many changing tables also come with shelves or drawers for easy access to baby clothing and diapers. You might prefer a portable changing table that is attached to a standard dresser. Look for changing tables with Velcro straps to prevent baby from rolling off.

## Nursery Themes

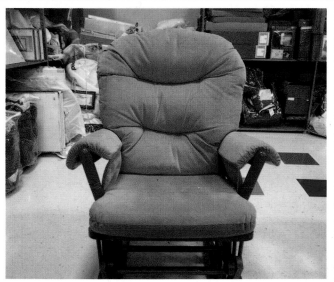

- Parents enjoy finding a theme for their nursery such as zoo or farm animals, Sesame Street, Winnie-the-Pooh, or Noah's ark are popular themes.

- The good thing about having a theme is that you can easily decorate your nursery with a variety of color shades and not just the traditional blue or pink.

- Plus, the themes themselves can grow with your baby well into preschool years if you convert the nursery a few years down the road.

### Co-Sleeping Dos and Don'ts

- Do not co-sleep on a water bed.

- Use a mesh guardrail to prevent baby from rolling out of bed.

- Place baby between guardrail and mother, not between parents.

- Use "back to sleep" positioning.

- Dress warmly with lightweight covers.

- Be sure the bed is large enough for the three of you and not too soft.

- Do not co-sleep if you are overtired.

- Avoid co-sleeping if you have had any alcohol or medications that make you sleepy.

- Do not co-sleep if you are obese or smoke in bed.

# BABY'S FIRST MOVEMENTS

## The first movements of the baby are often felt around sixteen to eighteen weeks of pregnancy

If you are like most mothers, those first identifiable baby kicks stop you dead in your tracks. You might think, "What was that?" It could be the first kicks of your baby. Around sixteen to eighteen weeks of pregnancy, most moms-to-be will feel those first few "kicks" from the baby, also known as "quickening."

Babies have all kinds of movements they can perform in utero in addition to kicking with their legs. They can roll over, yawn, stretch their arms and legs, and lift their head up. Your baby also has a startle reflex that you will be able to see when you place him on his back after he is born. It is not unusual to spot a baby on ultrasound sticking out her tongue or sucking on her fist.

*First Kicks*

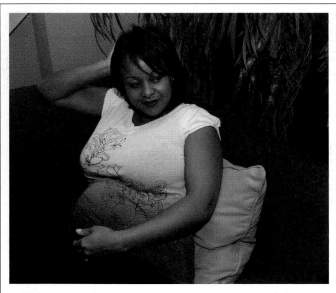

- Right around the time your baby is four months along, you may feel the first kicks.

- You might be surprised when the first kicks happen since you expected them to feel differently.

- By this time your baby weighs nearly half a pound and is about 5 inches in length.

- Don't forget to jot down the occasion of your first kicking sensation in your pregnancy journal or baby book!

*Personality*

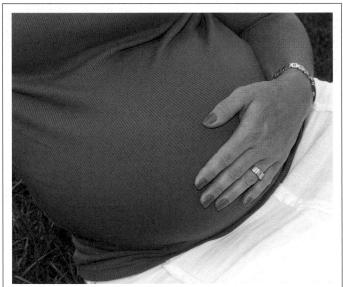

- So do you have a rocket scientist or a star athlete on the way?

- Some people think that the level of activity (or lack of activity) may give us a glimpse into the personalities of our babies.

- You may assume (incorrectly) that boys kick harder than girls.

- Perhaps the only thing our babies' kicks do tell us is that they are doing just fine.

Some studies show that a baby's movement increases significantly if the mother consumes a high-sugar drink. Believe it or not, your activity can affect your baby's movements. If you take a brisk walk, in essence you may be rocking your baby as your pelvis moves up and back with each step. When you lie down, your baby may decide to wake up and start moving more, once your activity level stops.

**ZOOM**

One of the ways you can distinguish hiccups from other baby movements is that they have a very small and rhythmic beat to them. Your baby does drink amniotic fluid, so it is not uncommon to feel your baby's hiccups from time to time toward the end of your second trimester and into your third trimester.

## *Sugar High*

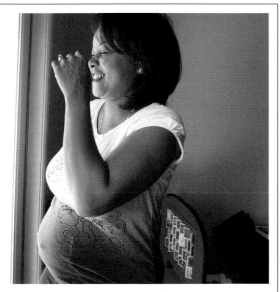

- It is no surprise that if mother eats or drinks something with tons of sugar, baby becomes more active in utero.

- Just ask any parent of a preschooler who has eaten too many sweets at their classmate's birthday party.

- Just remember to watch your own sugar intake during pregnancy as well as when your toddler begins to eat table foods.

- We all could benefit from watching our intake of sugar, no matter our age.

## *Rocking Your Baby*

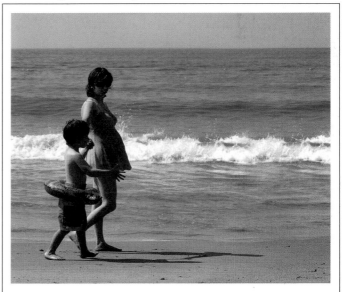

- When you are busy in your daily activities, going up and down stairs, walking, and staying active, it has the effect of rocking your baby to sleep.

- Knowing that movement calms your baby in utero, don't forget that the same movements will soothe your baby after he is born.

- Why do you think people naturally jostle a baby up and down when they are holding it?

- Your baby will love those movements to help him settle down to sleep.

# BABY'S IMMUNIZATIONS

## Immunization programs have greatly reduced the occurrence of many childhood diseases

As you meet and select your pediatrician in your second trimester, one of the things you should ask about is the current recommendations for childhood vaccinations, the recommended vaccine schedule in your area, and the vaccine requirements for daycare and school admissions in your municipality.

Immunizations contain part of the microorganism of the virus or bacteria and stimulate your baby's immune system to fight off the illness. Questions about the safety of immunizations and the risk from side effects have been raised periodically. Do some research while you are still pregnant and discuss your concerns with your pediatrician. That way

### Common Immunizations

- hepatitis A
- hepatitis B
- pneumococcal conjugate vaccine (PCV)
- DTaP (diphtheria, tetanus, acellular pertussis)
- Hib (meningitis)
- IPV (polio)
- influenza
- MMR (measles, mumps, rubella)
- varicella (chicken pox)
- MCV4 (bacterial meningitis)

### Reducing Fear

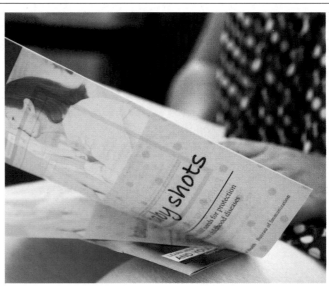

- Parents of newborns often react with great dismay at hearing their baby's pain cry at getting immunizations.

- Worse yet, older babies often recognize their surroundings and immediately start to cry in anticipation of getting shots.

- Some parents request that they hold their baby during administration of immunizations, to minimize the baby's distress.

- If you are breastfeeding, you may also ask to do this during the immunization, to help soothe and distract your baby.

you will have a plan and know what is in store for your first few pediatrician visits after the baby is born. Be informed consumers and know the risks and benefits of vaccinations before you make decisions.

Since several immunizations are combined, parents may request that they be given separately to reduce side effects. Others give a dose of infant acetaminophen before the vaccine to reduce the risk of fever. If you use acetaminophen for this purpose, your pediatrician can advise you on correct dosing. Many immunizations are mandatory for school.

············ YELLOW ● LIGHT ·············

Amid controversy that the preservative thimerosal, which was used in immunizations, was linked to autism, the AAP and the CDC requested that vaccine makers remove thimerosal from immunizations in 1999. Though there is no evidence to support this claim, if parents have concerns about this or other preservatives, they should discuss their concerns with their pediatrician.

## Keeping Records

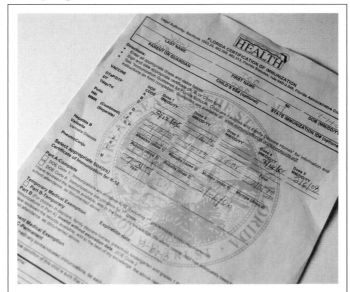

- Be sure to keep accurate records of your child's immunizations.

- Most pediatrician offices will give you a small booklet to bring to your baby's well visits to record the dates of each vaccine.

- Keep this booklet in a safe place with all of your important record-keeping so that you have access to it years later.

- It can be difficult to have to reconstruct your child's immunization records.

## Side Effects

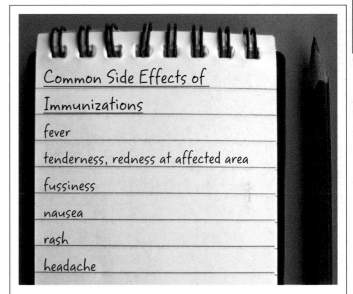

- Most babies seem to adjust well to vaccinations although some fussiness for a few hours is common.

- Taking the rest of the day for some quiet activity or a longer nap might help a baby who is feeling under the weather.

- Giving baby extra nursing and snuggle time is also a great idea.

- Be sure to contact your pediatrician if you have any concerns with symptoms your baby may have following an immunization.

# THE FOURTH MONTH

## Your baby's hand and foot prints begin to form in month four of your pregnancy

Your baby has grown quite a bit, and by the end of this month, she will be about 6 inches (15 to 16 centimeters) in length and will weigh nearly 8 1/2 ounces (250 grams). It's hard to imagine that as early as your fourth month of pregnancy, your baby's lungs and respiratory tract are already developing, including your baby's larynx, trachea, bronchi,

and lung buds. Even though your baby will not take his first breath until after birth, if you have an ultrasound this month, you might catch a glimpse of your baby "practicing" breathing movements.

Though it has been beating for many weeks, your baby's heart muscle becomes stronger in the fourth month. Sensory

**Highlights at Four Months**

- respiratory tract develops
- breathing movements detectable
- sensory organs differentiate
- hand and foot prints begin to form
- lanugo covers body

*Lanugo*

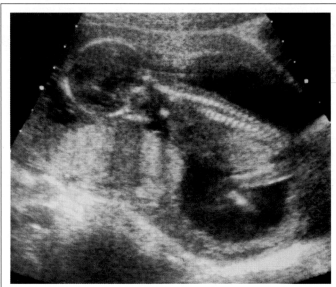

- The soft, downy body hair that grows on your baby during your pregnancy acts to regulate your baby's body temperature.

- Lanugo also provides insulation for your baby.

- If your baby is born right around your expected due date, parents will see very little lanugo left.

- The job of insulating baby has been taken over by layers of brown fat that develop at the end of pregnancy.

organs are beginning to differentiate, including his ears moving from his neck to his head, and his chin, nose, and forehead gradually becoming more defined.

Another new development is that the epidermal ridges on your baby's palms and feet start to form her unique hand and foot prints around the middle of the fourth month. The skin begins to lose its transparent look and become thicker now, and her arms and legs are growing longer than ever. Your baby's hair starts to grow on her head in the pattern of your own family's hairline.

**ZOOM**

Did you know that your uterus has an amazing filtering system? Your body completely replaces its supply of amniotic fluid with a unique filtering process every three to four hours. This is one way to make sure your baby is in a safe and clean environment.

## *Baby Footprints*

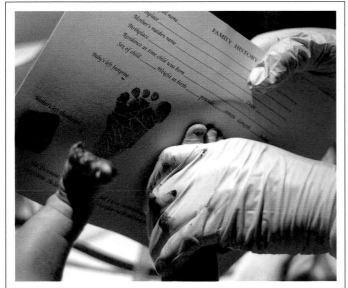

- Most birth settings record the baby's footprints for identification purposes.

- Parents may enjoy having another image made of their baby's footprint after birth to save.

- Fortunately footprints are made today with an inkless wipe on coated paper so it does not leave a mess.

- If you would like a copy of your baby's footprint as a keepsake, be sure to pack your baby book in your labor bag and take it to your place of birth.

## *Second Trimester Nutrition*

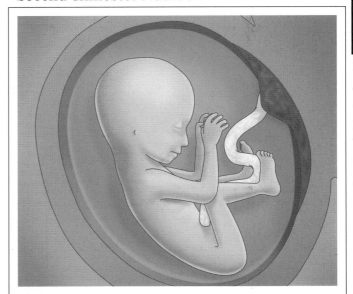

- Your second trimester nutrition is important as your baby continues to grow and develop.

- All of baby's organs that formed in the first trimester are now developing and growing new cells each week; be sure to add plenty of protein to each meal.

- Moms can become anemic easily during pregnancy so adding foods rich in iron will be important to your second trimester pregnancy diet.

- As your baby's body gets longer and his/her skeletal system grows, so does your need for calcium.

# THE FIFTH MONTH

## Your baby reaches the one-pound mark during month five of your pregnancy

By five months your baby's development is well under way. His sense of hearing is well developed by the fifth month, and we know that babies at this stage will respond to noises outside the mother's body. Don't forget to take advantage of your baby's ability to hear by talking and/or reading to your baby whenever possible.

From week twenty to week twenty-four of pregnancy, your baby's teeth begin to grow their layers of enamel, which is the outermost layer of the teeth, as well as the dentin, which is the layer that sits just below the tooth enamel. Research also shows that your baby is able to distinguish taste as early as the fifth month of pregnancy.

### Highlights at Five Months

- sense of hearing develops
- enamel and dentin layers form on teeth
- sense of taste develops
- colon expands
- testes descend in males
- baby reaches one-pound mark in weight

### *Familiar Sounds*

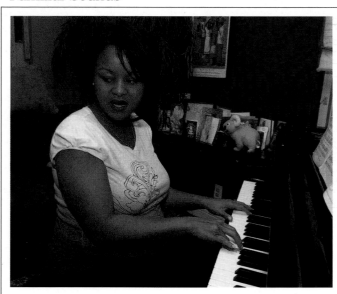

- Your baby's sense of hearing is already developed by the fifth month of pregnancy.

- This means that all of the sounds in your environment, like busy city streets and dogs barking, can be heard.

- Voices of family members will already be familiar to your baby after he is born since he has been able to hear them from your second trimester.

- You can expose your baby to some of the wonderful sounds in his environment, such as music.

Other changes in the fifth month of pregnancy include your baby's colon growing longer and expanding upward into her abdomen. If you are carrying a boy, there are already changes happening in his reproductive system. As early as the fifth month, his testes will begin to descend.

If you are keeping track of your baby's weight each month, make a note that your baby is likely to be right around one pound at this time. With four months to go, expect that your baby will gain seven times that amount by the time you give birth.

Both mom and baby are growing more hair! Your baby is growing its fine body hair, called lanugo. Meanwhile, some moms find that the hair on their head becomes thicker and on top of that, they notice hair growing in all sorts of unusual places! The baby's fine lanugo does disappear in late pregnancy, but sometimes mom's coarse hair growth may not go away quite so easily.

## Sweet Tooth

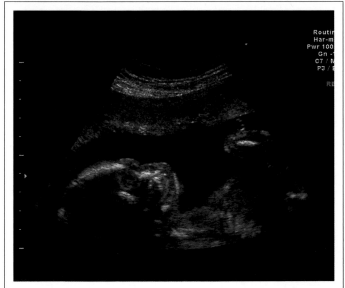

- Scientists have revealed that babies have taste abilities at five months of pregnancy.

- German researchers added a sweetener to the amniotic fluid in the uterus.

- The added sweetener caused human babies to swallow twice as fast.

- So it's not a surprise that we prefer sweets even before we are born, all the more reasons to be careful of over-doing it on this powerful substance.

## Baby's Size

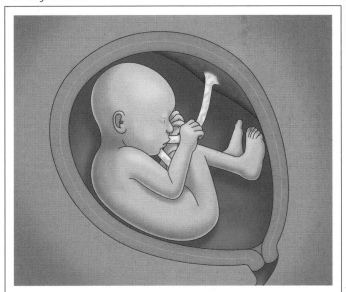

- Even though your baby's body becomes more proportioned right about now, she is still very lean with long legs and arms but no body fat.

- As you finish up your fifth month of pregnancy, your baby will be about 8 inches (20 centimeters) long.

- You might feel as if your baby should be heavier by looking at your own weight gain!

- Yet she typically weighs around 1 pound (500 grams) by week twenty-three of pregnancy.

# THE SIXTH MONTH

## The "baby fat" layers help to prepare your little one for life outside your uterus

It's hard to imagine that you only have sixteen weeks of pregnancy left! All the while, your baby will be growing and changing each and every week. Early in your sixth month, the thick, cheesy coating that will eventually cover your baby's body starts to form. This coating, called vernix, acts as a "Scotchgard" to protect your baby's skin from the surrounding amniotic fluid for many months.

Another big change is that your baby's bronchioles and bronchi are expanding into her lungs this month and even her nostrils begin to open. Your baby's eyes have reached the point where they are completely developed, even though they do not open yet.

*Highlights at Six Months*

- vernix forms
- bronchioles and bronchi expand
- eyes are completely developed
- meconium appears
- layers of brown fat form

*Vernix*

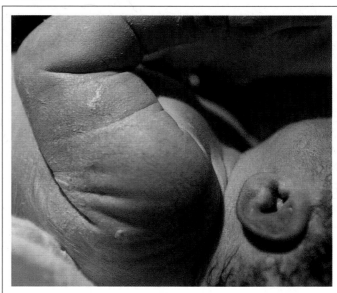

- Your baby's sebaceous glands produce vernix caseosa to protect her skin during pregnancy.

- This substance is a thick, cheesy coating that forms during the second trimester but diminishes until late pregnancy where you might see it only in folds.

- Vernix is made up of oil from the baby's skin cells that have already sloughed off her body.

- Some experts believe that vernix may also have an antibacterial component, so maybe it helps to protect her against infection as well.

The very first appearance of meconium occurs in your sixth month. Meconium is the stool that your baby produces while in utero and will begin to pass for the first few days of life. Since your baby is not digesting food, this dark tarlike stool is nearly sterile and is made up of amniotic fluid, lanugo, bile, and mucous.

In your sixth month your baby is starting to add layers of brown fat. This fat accumulates in the baby's back, upper spine, and shoulders, and will help him regulate his body temperature after he is born and help to prevent hypothermia.

········· YELLOW ● LIGHT ··········

If your water breaks in labor and the fluid is dark yellow to greenish in color, it is likely a sign that your baby is passing meconium into the amniotic fluid. This happens in about 5 to 10 percent of births. As a result, your care provider will need to suction your baby's airway to remove as much meconium as possible before your baby begins to breathe.

## Brown Fat

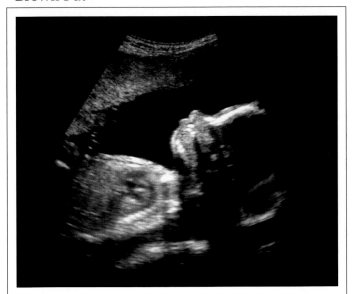

- Just like you put on your winter coat when the temperature outside is cold, your baby adds layers of brown fat to help keep her warm.

- When she leaves her toasty environment of your uterus and enters the much colder outside environment, she will need this extra layer of fat.

- This is an important regulator for your baby to maintain her body temperature.

- After she is born, placing her on mother's chest with a warm blanket is another way to keep her warm.

## Baby's Brain/Nervous System

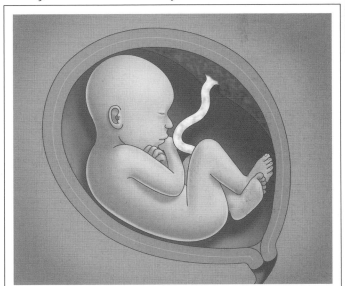

- You might be surprised to learn that your baby's brain is still developing.

- The cerebral cortex in your baby's brain adds new layers in the sixth month.

- Your baby's nerve cells have been dividing to form new ones. That process taking place in your baby's nervous system ends by week twenty-four.

- This is a great time to be reminded about good eating habits to help grow your baby's brain.

# YOUR THIRD-TRIMESTER CHECKLIST

## Mothers complete childbirth classes and practice labor techniques in the last trimester

Before you know it, you will be winding down to the last thirteen weeks of pregnancy. If you are working full-time, you should be making a plan for your maternity leave and when to leave work. Some mothers find it easier to take a few weeks at the end of their pregnancy to slow down, rest up, and get those last few items checked off their checklist. If your maternity leave is limited, you may prefer to work right up until the time you go into labor.

Your last trimester is notorious for being the most tiring and the most uncomfortable. Carrying all of the additional weight from the baby might wear you out during the day as well as make it harder to get comfortable sleep at night. During the

### Third-Trimester Checklist

- Complete your childbirth class and any other classes.
- Complete your birth plan.
- Practice techniques learned in class.
- Finish additional reading on birth or parenting issues.
- Complete baby nursery or shopping for baby items.
- Make arrangements for pets or older children when you are in labor.
- Begin perineal massage at thirty-four weeks.

### Research Tips

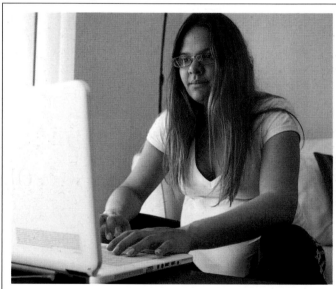

- The Internet can be a useful resource for expectant parents.

- Many Web sites contain helpful tips and research-based information.

- Make sure the advice you are getting comes from a recognized Web site.

- Advice can be misleading or inaccurate if it comes from a personal blog or a chat room.

day, you might be plagued by many other discomforts such as heartburn, constipation, and frequent urination. All of these changes take their toll and you may simply be unable to keep up the pace you were used to in the previous few months. Listen to your body and rest when you need it!

Make sure you are using these last few weeks to research your options regarding birth planning. You will learn new techniques in your childbirth classes such as massage, breathing patterns, and relaxation exercises. Set aside several times each week for review and practice.

## Staying Cool

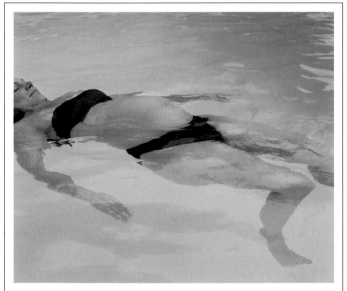

- Progesterone can cause an increase in your body temperature by about 0.9 degrees F.

- Not to mention you have your own heat source now!

- Taking cool showers, and swimming can also help cool you down.

- Wear fabrics that are lighter and help your body release heat, such as cotton.

## Reduce Swelling

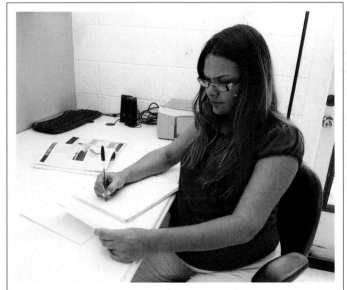

- It is not uncommon to see swelling in late pregnancy in your ankles and fingers.

- Continue to drink plenty of fluids—at least eight to ten glasses of water a day.

- Try to avoid standing for long periods of time.

- Keep moving throughout the day with regular stretching exercises.

3RD TRIMESTER: MOM

# LATE-PREGNANCY EMOTIONS

## Mood swings and insomnia go hand in hand with the last few months of pregnancy

Hormonal surges during pregnancy can wreak havoc with your emotions. Let your husband and family know that this is all a part of pregnancy and you are not losing your mind. Being supported and validated for those up-and-down emotions is vital during your remaining weeks. Moms also complain that they have trouble sleeping for multiple reasons. Not only is it

a struggle to get comfortable, but the frequent trips to the bathroom disrupt what little sleep you are getting. On top of that, you might notice that your sleep is filled with disturbing and vivid dreams. While we don't know the exact reason behind the more frequent strange dreams or nightmares, it only makes sense that your mind is full of anticipation for

### Role of Estrogen

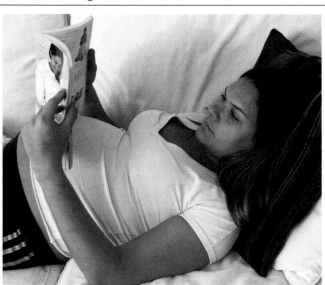

- In addition to causing mood swings, estrogen plays an instrumental role in pregnancy.

- Estrogen helps to increase the blood flow in the uterus.

- It also helps to maintain your pregnancy and stimu-

lates your baby to grow and mature.

- Estrogen, in combination with relaxin, helps to relax your pelvic joints and ligaments and even increases the flexibility of your nipples to help prepare you for breastfeeding.

### Pregnancy Dreams

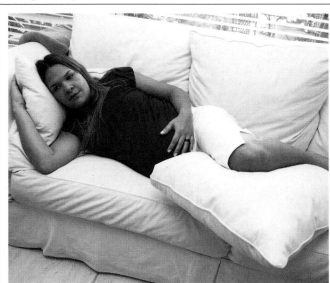

- Dreams are a way that our brain tries to sort out fears and concerns, and finish undone business.

- Keep a pen and notebook near your bedside to jot down your dreams. Is there anything symbolic about your dream images?

- What does your dream reveal about any hidden fears you might be suppressing?

- Share your dream with your partner or a trusted friend to see what advice they can offer you.

the future, your hormones are surging, and the challenges of pregnancy can add to your stress. You might find journaling or talking to a friend about your unusual dreams helpful.

Settling down with a consistent routine at the same time every night might help you shut off your busy brain. If you are not bothered by heartburn, try eating a small snack (such as fruit slices or carrot sticks) before bed. Turn off the TV and take a warm bath. Right before bed is also an ideal time to practice your relaxation exercises with your partner.

One piece of advice for expectant mothers is to remember not to worry about little things. If your baby comes early and you never finish the final coat of paint in your nursery, your baby will never notice. Most likely, the only person who will be concerned about the lack of paint will be you.

## White Noise

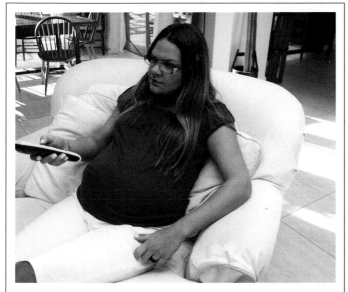

- A great sleep aid to block out excessive noise is the use of a white-noise machine.

- White-noise machines also help babies sleep better since they are already used to the noise level in your uterus!

- These can be purchased at many department stores and baby stores.

- Manufacturers recommend setting the volume of noise low to begin with to help your ears adjust.

Tips for Restful Sleep

- Take a bath before bed.

- Try eating a light snack.

- Do not watch TV in your bedroom.

- Keep your room as dark as possible.

- Use a white-noise machine or fan.

- If you wake up, don't look at the clock.

- Keep your bedtime routines consistent.

# MANAGING DISCOMFORTS
## One of the most common physical complaints of late pregnancy is back pain

At some point in your last few weeks of pregnancy, you will be quite ready to give birth. Of course you will be ready to meet your baby, but often the motivating factor behind your urgency is to finally get relief from your discomforts.

Back pain is one of the most common complaints of late pregnancy. Your body will tend to balance the extra weight of the baby by drawing back your shoulders and moving your pelvis forward—thus the pregnancy waddle! Babies who tend to favor a posterior position (with the back of their head against your back) also contribute to late pregnancy back pain. Doing pelvic tilts and visiting a chiropractor familiar with issues of pregnancy can be a tremendous help.

### Back Pain Relief

- pelvic tilts (angry cat)
- sitting on a birth ball
- warm compresses
- chiropractic care
- side-lying position with leg-wedge pillow between knees
- using a body pillow for sleeping comfort

### Birth Ball for Comfort

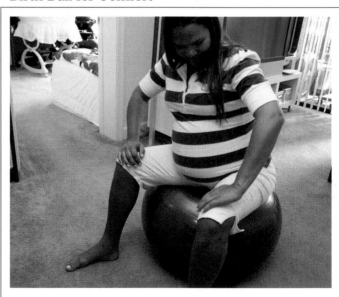

- Many mothers find that birth balls are more comfortable than sitting in a chair during late pregnancy.

- Sitting on a birth ball relaxes your pelvic floor muscles and can strengthen the muscles in your lower back.

- They also help improve your posture and can reduce shortness-of-breath symptoms.

- It helps to become more comfortable sitting on a ball during your pregnancy so that it will be a familiar tool during labor.

Some moms might find that using a birth ball can reduce back pain.

Digestive upsets also top the discomfort list of late pregnancy. Indigestion and heartburn occur when your stomach gets pushed up by your expanding uterus. Eating smaller meals and trying soothing herbs such as chamomile tea can help digestive upsets. Constipation is common since your smooth muscles relax during pregnancy. You might find getting plenty of fiber, drinking more water, and exercising can relieve constipation.

## Chamomile for Digestion

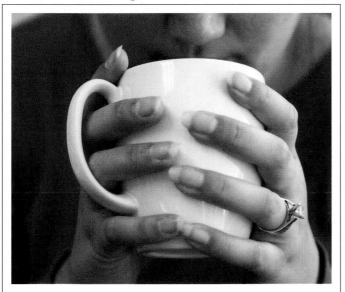

- Chamomile is a popular herb to help with late pregnancy heartburn and digestive upsets.

- It contains an anti-inflammatory ingredient that reduces inflammation in the digestive tract.

- Drinking a cup of chamomile tea in the morning is a popular aid for a sore stomach.

- Chamomile is not recommended for mothers in their first trimester or for mothers who have allergies to ragweed.

## Relief

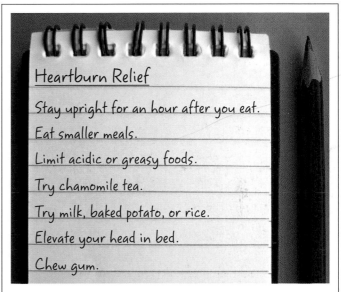

Heartburn Relief

Stay upright for an hour after you eat.

Eat smaller meals.

Limit acidic or greasy foods.

Try chamomile tea.

Try milk, baked potato, or rice.

Elevate your head in bed.

Chew gum.

- Heartburn is a frequent complaint among mothers in late pregnancy.

- As your baby grows, the uterus expands and compresses your stomach pushing up stomach contents.

- The valve in your esophagus also relaxes, allowing stomach acid to seep upward, causing heartburn.

- Treatments can help, but symptoms often lessen after your baby settles lower into your pelvis in the last weeks of pregnancy.

# BABY-PROOFING YOUR HOME

## Use baby gates at the top and bottom of stairwells to make your home safer for baby

Unless you have done a thorough baby-proofing of your house already, now is the time to make sure it is not an obstacle course of unsafe zones.

You can start the baby-proofing process by crawling around your home and looking at the places within your reach. Electrical outlets can be covered and all lower cabinets should have locks. Cleaning products can be moved to higher cabinets. Watch for hanging cords from lamps and other appliances. Put away any loose items or knickknacks on tables. You may want to look for several baby gates on sale now so that you can put them up at the top and bottom of stairways as soon as your baby becomes mobile.

### Safety Checklist

- Cover outlets.
- Lock cabinets.
- Move cleaning products.
- Tuck away hanging cords.
- Put away loose items.
- Use baby gates.
- Adjust temperature of hot water heater.
- Install smoke detectors.
- Put fence around outdoor pool.
- Anchor heavy furniture or appliances to the wall.

### Out of Reach

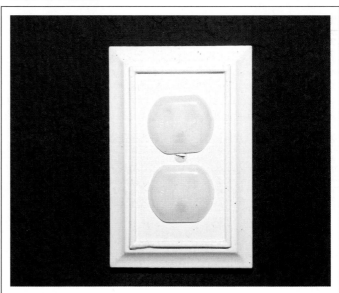

- It is only a matter of months before your baby will be investigating everything that is at his eye level in your home.

- Outlet covers are easy to use and can be found in grocery or hardware stores.

- Cabinet locks are quick to install and only cost about $2 each.

- Any toxic or hazardous cleaning products should be moved to cabinets that are at parents' eye level.

Sometimes the corners of tables, beds, chairs, and desks can have sharp edges. Consider replacing them in the areas where your baby will be playing, or look for plastic safety bumpers for all furniture with sharp corners. Adjust the temperature of your hot water heater to 120 degrees F to avoid burns. Be sure you have several smoke detectors installed in your home and at least one fire extinguisher. If you have a backyard pool, make sure to have a secured and locked fence installed all the way around.

## Preventing Burns

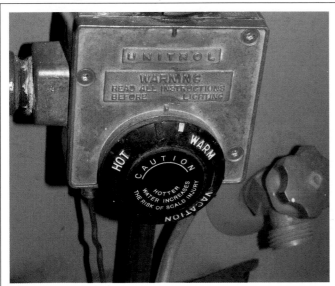

- Burns in the home are one of the most common childhood injuries.

- Turn down the hot water heater to prevent accidental burns.

- Place a cover over the metal spout in the bathroom tub to avoid burns during bathing.

- When you are cooking, turn handles of pots and pans inward toward the middle of the stove.

## Smoke Detectors

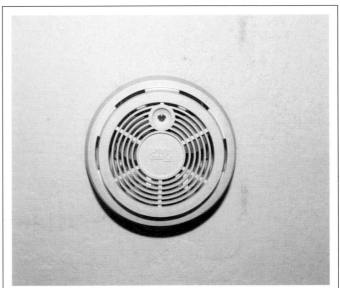

- Install a smoke detector in your home and test it every month.

- The batteries should be replaced when you change your clocks, or replaced twice a year, or ten years for a lithium-type battery.

- Costs run about $25 to $30 for a standard battery-operated smoke detector.

- Newer models include a photoelectric detector that allows parents to record a message in their own voice as opposed to sounding an alarm.

3RD TRIMESTER: MOM

# BABY'S POSITION

## Mothers can encourage their babies into a more favorable position for birth in late pregnancy

When your baby is in a posterior position, the back of her head is facing your back. While there is no way for you to identify your baby's position for certain unless your care provider does an ultrasound, there are some symptoms that might make you suspicious. If your labor is taking longer and there is a period of time without progress, it could mean your

baby needs to get into a more favorable position. Having a significant amount of your pain in your back is another possible indicator of a posterior baby.

So is having a posterior baby harmful? No, not at all: During labor, most babies cooperate nicely and turn before they are born. A few (3 percent) even decide to be born "sunny side

### My Baby Could be Posterior When:

- baby's heartbeat is difficult to find or far to the mother's left.

- mother has more pubic bone discomfort.

- mother has a slowly progressing labor

- mother has significant back pain with contractions

*Side-lying Position*

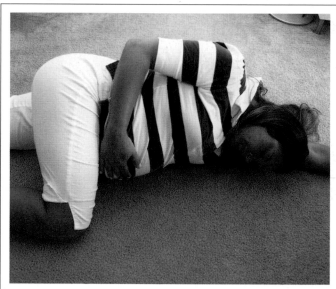

- Lying on your side can help turn a posterior baby during pregnancy and childbirth.

- Gravity can help to pull the back of your baby's head to the front of your pelvis.

- Lie down on the opposite side of where the baby's back is positioned.

- Be sure your top knee is nearly touching your belly and your lower leg is straight.

up." But sometimes if your baby stays in a posterior position during labor, it can make your labor longer and more difficult. Posterior babies are notorious for causing "back labor," with back pain both during and in between contractions.

While some experts have a "wait and see" approach and recommend positions to turn a posterior baby while a mother is in labor, a newer idea is to prevent babies from staying put in this position in the last weeks. For example, if you sit in a recliner, gravity will tend to pull the heaviest part of your baby (the back of your baby's head) toward your back or into a posterior position. However, positions such as on your hands and knees can bring the back of your baby's head around to an anterior position. Using various positions such as a side-lying lunge, sitting backwards in a chair without arms, or straddling a birth ball frequently in the last few weeks of pregnancy can help to keep your baby from staying in a posterior position.

## Hands and Knees

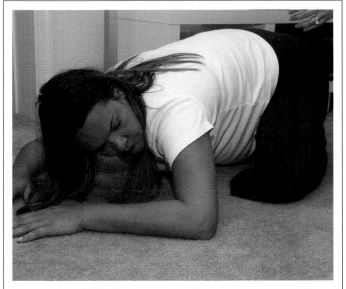

- An easy and effective position to turn a baby is a hands and knees position.

- This position also works great to reduce back pain during pregnancy and labor.

- You can lean over on the seat of a chair, using a pillow for support, or lean over a birth ball.

- A good rule of thumb is to use this position during pregnancy or labor when your back is hurting.

## Turning Baby

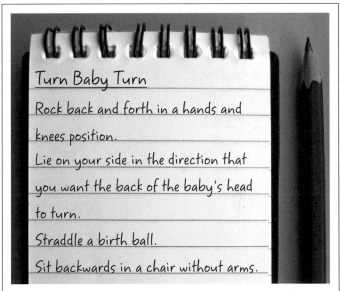

Turn Baby Turn

Rock back and forth in a hands and knees position.

Lie on your side in the direction that you want the back of the baby's head to turn.

Straddle a birth ball.

Sit backwards in a chair without arms.

- Laboring with a baby in a posterior position can be a difficult way to give birth.

- Women often report that they had trouble finding relief from the back labor associated with a posterior baby.

- Keep in mind that most babies do turn with some extra time, patience and position changes.

- If not, your baby may simply decide to come into the world by taking the "scenic route."

# LABOR TIPS FOR DADS

## Mothers enjoy massage and practicing relaxation exercises in the last weeks of pregnancy

Fathers today are taking a much more active role than their fathers or grandfathers did in preparation for birth. Dad's role becomes even more important in the last few weeks as preparations for baby are well under way, mom becomes tired and uncomfortable, and childbirth is right around the corner.

With all of the methods and techniques out there, fathers may wonder what really does work during labor. The truth is that dads have a heads-up in this department. You already know what she likes and doesn't like when she is in pain, and how to comfort her when she is stressed or cannot cope well. Mom is not likely to cope with pain in labor using techniques

### *Massage*

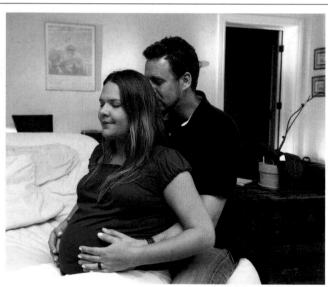

- Massage is one of the ways to increase the level of oxytocin, the "love hormone."

- Massage also helps to loosen mother's tired muscles and relieves aches from pregnancy discomforts.

- Find out what kinds of massage mom needs or likes— firm pressure, light stroking, or deep kneading.

- You might consider taking a couples' massage class if this topic is not covered in your childbirth class.

### *Music*

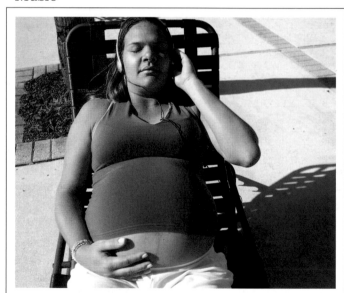

- If you like to have music playing in the background while you are at home, chances are that you will also find it relaxing during labor.

- Music is a perfect addition to enhance massage techniques or deep relaxation.

- Have a variety of music to listen to for various stages of labor.

- Soothing, gentle music is perfect for relaxation, and stronger, louder rhythms work better to give you an energy boost.

that are completely foreign to her. Some of the top techniques to practice include deep breathing in conjunction with relaxation. Mothers might also like a firm massage or a stroking massage during or in between contractions.

You might bring massage oils or lotions that you have already used during your relaxation practice. Practicing the techniques you are both learning in class is the only way for you, as the primary labor partner, to feel confident in using them during labor. Many mothers find that music is helpful, so you could make a CD of her favorite music to play during labor.

## MAKE IT EASY

Roving Body Check: This method was created by Penny Simkin. As Mom slowly breathes, her labor partner places his hands on a body part and presses in lightly as she inhales, releasing slowly as she exhales. He continues down her body, focusing on a different part with each breath. She focuses on her partner's touch with inhalation and relaxes on her exhalation.

### Take-Charge Routine by Penny Simkin

- Remain calm with a firm touch and encouraging voice.

- Stay close to her, your face near hers.

- Anchor her, holding her shoulders or her head in your hands.

- Make eye contact, tell her to look at you.

- Try a different breathing pattern or ritual during labor.

- Encourage her to breathe with you.

- Talk to her in between contractions; repeat yourself.

- Use this method any time mother is having trouble coping.

### What If She Says She Can't Go On?

- Don't give up on her.

- Ask for additional help from care providers if you need it.

- Remind her of the baby.

- Remember her prior wishes regarding pain medication.

- How quickly is her labor progressing?

- How much further does she still need to go?

- How does she respond to your coaching?

- Respect her wishes even if she changes her mind.

# BABY NAMES

## When selecting a name for your baby, choose one that will grow with your child

What should you consider when you are naming your baby? Using first or last names from your families is a common way to select names today. Parents may choose family names as their baby name. It is not uncommon to see the mother's maiden name used as a middle name as a way to carry on her family name.

There is a downside to choosing a popular name for your baby. If you like that name, so do many other parents. Your son or daughter is likely to share that name with several others in their class. Be sensitive to the fact that having a popular name may make it harder for your child to find his or her own individuality.

*Choosing Names*

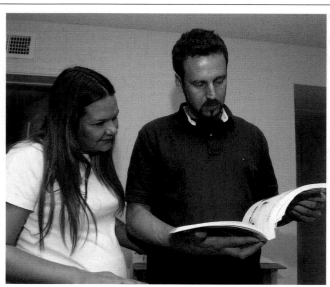

- If you are having difficulty agreeing on names, here's a suggestion:

- Have both mom and dad select their top ten boy or girl names using books, Web sites, and any other resource.

- Write them down on a piece of paper and then swap lists.

- Find at least two names from each person's list that you could agree to.

*Family Names*

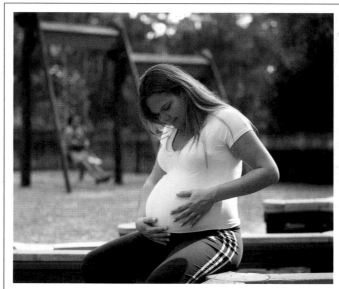

- Choosing a family name is often done for tradition or to remember a loved one who has passed on.

- A common way to pass down a name that belongs to a special person is to use it as your child's middle name.

- Some parents might combine a family name with a different name to make it a bit more unique.

- Two examples of this could be combining the name Mary and Louise into Marylou or Steven and Nash becomes Stash.

Another thing to consider is choosing a name that will "grow" with your child as she gets older. Names that sound perfect for a five-year-old girl may not be suitable for a sixty-year-old woman. While most of the time, selecting the right name for your baby is fun, it can be challenging. What if one of you is attached to a name that the other person has a negative association with? Learning ways to compromise or agree on a completely different name may be in order. The good thing is that there are millions of names to choose from, so enjoy your search in finding just the right name for your baby.

Parents may want to choose names with special meaning in their search for a baby name. For example, Michael, a name that is often in the top ten list for boys is a Hebrew name and means "Who is like God". One of the tried-and-true girl's names, Hannah, means "favored grace." It can be fun to discover what your favorite baby names mean.

## Expressing Individuality

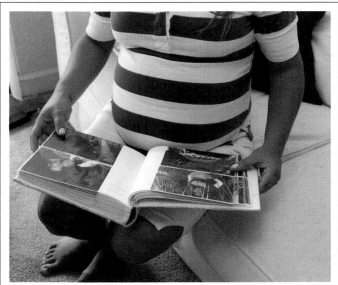

- You might decide to have several baby names "ready to go" and then wait until meeting your baby before you decide.

- It might be hard to imagine that your baby's personality emerges during the first few days after birth.

- However, you will soon see that one of the names you selected is a much better fit than others you had considered.

- Some parents may need a few days to try on a few names for size before they find the right one.

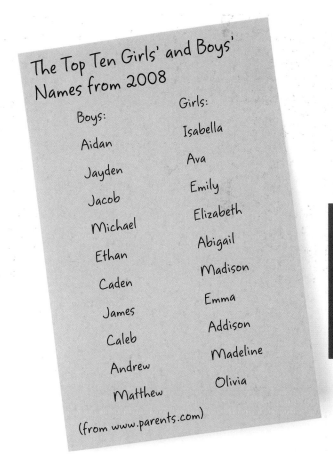

The Top Ten Girls' and Boys' Names from 2008

Boys:
Aidan
Jayden
Jacob
Michael
Ethan
Caden
James
Caleb
Andrew
Matthew

Girls:
Isabella
Ava
Emily
Elizabeth
Abigail
Madison
Emma
Addison
Madeline
Olivia

(from www.parents.com)

# YOUR BABY SHOWER

## Baby showers give friends and family the perfect opportunity to help mom and dad with expensive baby items

The last trimester is the time when friends and family begin to plan your baby shower. If you are involved in the preparations or if your party planners need some ideas, here are a few to help get you started.

Discount party stores are just the right place to find invitations, decorations, and paper goods. When you send out invitations, be sure to let your guests know where they can access your baby registry. Showers are the perfect time to request those large items like strollers or car seats, where multiple party guests can pool their resources to purchase them.

You cannot attend a bridal or baby shower these days without playing a few games. Everyone loves fun, competitive

### Shower Game: Who Knows Mom Best?

Write down several questions ahead of time such as:

- gender of the baby

- due date

- when baby was conceived

- one book the mother has read

- where the mother plans to have the baby

- who will be there at the birth

Read questions out loud to group. Each person writes down her own answers. The person who gets the most number of answers correct wins a prize.

### Remember the Baby Items

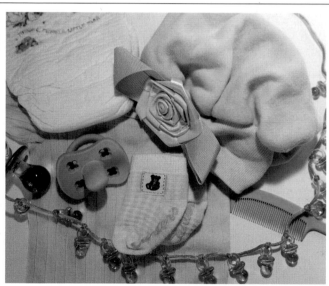

- For another game idea, place a tray out with small baby items on it such as a bottle, diaper pin, pacifier, bib, baby spoon, etc.

- Leave the tray out for about thirty seconds for your guests to look at without making any notes.

- Give your guests ten minutes to jot down as many baby items as they can remember.

- The person who remembers the most items on the tray wins a prize.

games where there are prizes given to winners. Make sure you have a few extra prizes ready, just in case you have two or three winners in each game!

Since baby showers often take place over a lunch hour, make sure to have a platter of fresh fruits or vegetables available in addition to your other party foods. Check with your guests ahead of time to see if anyone has allergies or a special diet. Shower guests might also enjoy a range of beverages such as punch, water, coffee, and tea. Baby showers are not just an opportunity to socialize, but help moms feel supported.

*Party Foods*

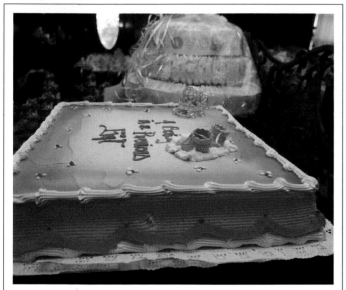

- To make food preparations easier for your party planners, select a theme for your baby shower party foods.

- Some ideas for themes include "Picnic Lunch," "Mexican," or "Desserts."

- Ask each guest to contribute a food item that goes along with that theme. Keep a record of what everyone is bringing to avoid duplication.

- Not only is that a great way to divide the responsibilities, but it allows for some creativity from your guests.

*Baby Shower Checklist*

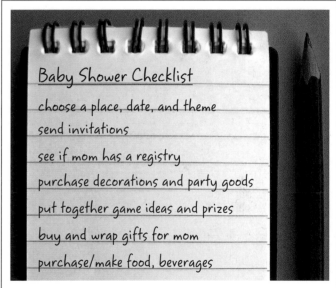

- Everyone loves attending a party, especially something as exciting as a baby shower.

- Baby showers, like most gatherings can be a ton of preparation so encourage your friends and family to work together to divide up the responsibilities.

- In addition to the pre-party jobs, make sure you have a designated person to keep track of gifts and where to send those thank-you notes.

- Most importantly, have a great time with your friends and family!

159

# PREPARING SIBLINGS FOR BABY

## Help with sibling adjustment by including the baby's brother or sister in baby-care activities

It can be a rude awakening for an older sibling to find out that this new baby will not be returning to the hospital! When you bring your second or later baby home, you can expect there will be some adjustment required for everyone in the family.

A typical two- or three-year-old, and sometimes older children, will react negatively to having to share your love and attention with a new baby. Sometimes the older child's behavior will include more frequent temper tantrums and "testing" behaviors.

Keeping your routines consistent, including bedtimes, mealtimes, and activities (such as preschool and playgroups), will be important for your older child. Whenever possible,

### Tips on Sibling Adjustment

- Keep your older child's routines consistent.

- Stick to your established rules.

- Expect testing behaviors.

- Include siblings in baby-care activities.

- Delay major changes.

### Regression Is Normal

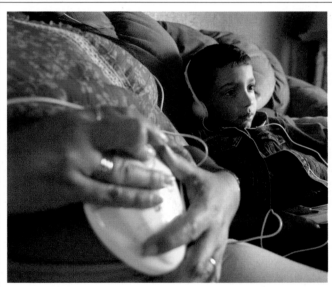

- A sibling is told repeatedly that she/he is now a "big" sister or brother.

- Unfortunately this is not always received as a compliment and it may even be a threat.

- You might be surprised that your older child regresses and wants to "be a baby."

- Instead, try to emphasize all of the great things he/she can do that the baby cannot.

include the child in activities with the new baby. You can ask the older sibling to bring you bath items or diapers and emphasize "what a great helper you are!" If you are feeding your baby, ask your older child to bring over a book so you can read it together. Try not to make any major changes, such as moving to a new room or potty training, within a few months before or after the baby arrives.

This period of adjustment is hard for parents and family. But there is good news. Children who have younger siblings at home are better adjusted when they enter kindergarten.

## Importance of Routines

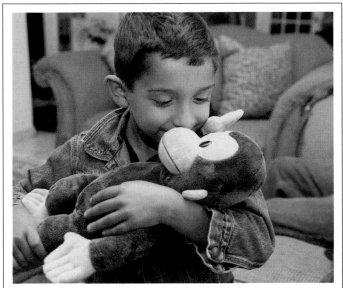

- When the new baby arrives, it feels like everything has changed in the sibling's world.

- It will be important for the sibling's routines to remain the same.

- Hold off on taking him out of a crib, moving him to a new room, potty-training or making any major changes in his routine until several months after the baby is born.

- Try to stick to the routines your child is used to, including preschool, day care, or daytime activities.

## Healthy Parenting

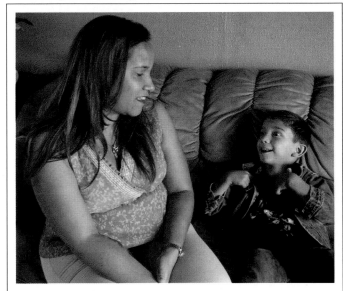

- You might feel so sorry for your older child and the adjustment he needs to make that you're tempted to make exceptions to your rules in the home.

- Part of your parenting involves lovingly sticking to those boundaries, despite outbursts or temper tantrums.

- If you do not budge from these rules, your child will see you as an authority.

- Ultimately it will also be a much healthier dynamic for the entire family.

# THE SEVENTH MONTH

## At seven months your baby is preparing for birth by moving his head down into your pelvis

This is an exciting time for your baby as you move into your last trimester. Changes are continuing to take place with your baby every week! At the beginning of your seventh month, your baby's fingernails and toenails are fully formed and your baby's body is more lean and less wrinkled and red in appearance. Around twenty-eight weeks the hair on your baby's head is growing longer than the lanugo on her body. Though you wouldn't be able to see them yet, all of your baby's permanent teeth are now present!

There are several changes happening with your baby's eyes this month. She can open her eyes and even the retinal layers (which are the inner part of the eye that respond to light)

Highlights at Seven Months

• fingernails and toenails have developed

• body less wrinkled

• hair on head grows

• eyes open and pupils dilate

• moves in unison with mother's speech

• becomes vertex

*Baby's Eyes*

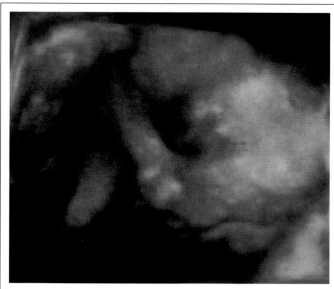

- Do you wonder what color your baby's eyes will be?

- If your baby's eyes change, they will likely do so within the first six to nine months after birth.

- If your baby was born with blue eyes, they may darken over time to brown, green, or hazel.

- However, if your baby is born with brown eyes, they will likely stay brown.

are completing their development. Her pupils can also dilate now in response to light.

Researchers have noticed that babies can move in rhythm to their mother's speech as early as six to seven months of pregnancy. This is one way that your baby is becoming prepared for the intonation and inflection of language. As your baby begins preparations for birth, he moves his head down into your pelvis. This head-down position is called vertex. If this is not your first baby, he may not be vertex as early in your pregnancy, but by late pregnancy or labor, he will be.

## Early Language Development

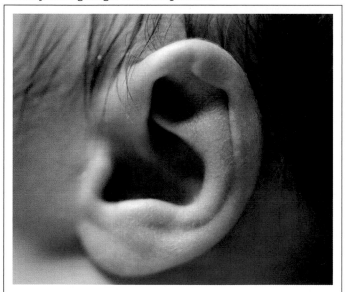

- Even in the last three to four months of pregnancy, your baby is already learning language.

- Your baby will be able to hear your voice as well as sounds outside the uterus.

- When the inflection of your voice changes as you speak, your baby is already beginning to learn those inflections.

- Researchers have seen babies in utero and even in the first days of life move their bodies in synchrony to the rhythms of the mother's speech.

## Baby's Position

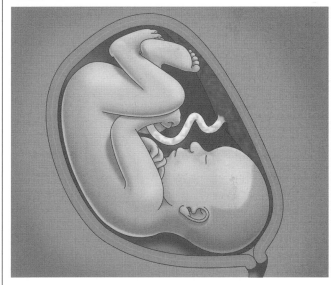

- Your baby can be in many positions in your pelvis in the last trimester.

- About 5 percent of babies are in breech positions, including frank breech (buttocks first), footling breech (feet first), or complete breech (sitting cross-legged).

- Babies can also lay sideways across your pelvis, known as a transverse lie.

- The most common (and easiest for birth) is vertex, which means your baby's head presents first into your pelvis.

# THE EIGHTH MONTH

## The baby's earliest signs of having REM sleep are in month eight of pregnancy

Are your maternity clothes fitting more snugly now? There is good reason for that. Your baby reaches about 5 pounds and nearly 13 inches in length by the end of this month. Experts have discovered that babies are capable of REM (rapid eye movement) sleep as early as thirty-two weeks of pregnancy. This means that your little one is already dreaming in her sleep.

The amount of amniotic fluid in your baby's sac is now at its peak. Don't forget that your baby swallows this fluid and is practicing breathing movements while in your uterus. In addition, your baby begins to add a layer of subcutaneous fat under her skin this month. This fat layer provides insulation for your baby to stay warm after she is born.

### Highlights at Eight Months

- baby reaches five pounds
- REM sleep
- additional subcutaneous fat layer
- bones growing longer

### Brain Power

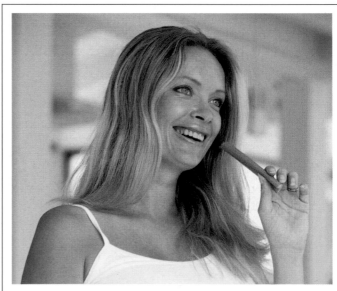

- You might assume that your baby's brain development was completed in the first trimester.

- The truth is that your baby's brain is still growing new cells and developing well into your last trimester.

- One of the changes in this last part of pregnancy involves the separation of the two hemispheres of the baby's brain.

- This is a crucial time to be getting good nutrition and avoiding exposure to harmful substances.

You might be tempted to cut back if your weight gain is on the high side, but no matter where your weight is, do not cut back on good nutrition. Your baby's bones are growing rapidly in the entire third trimester, so grab some extra calcium with meals and snacks. Even your baby's brain continues to grow new brain cells during the last trimester, and as a result, you and your baby will both need adequate protein.

## Fat Layers

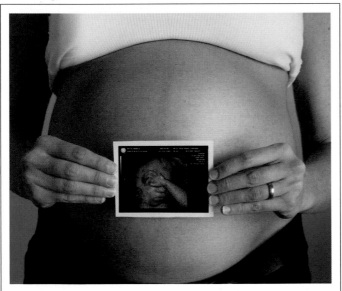

- Subcutaneous fat is added in month eight of pregnancy.

- It is an additional fat layer just below your baby's skin.

- If your baby is born this month, your baby will look long and lean to you, since you will not see much of this fat yet.

- If your baby arrives closer to your due date, he/she will have several more weeks to build up a generous amount of these fat layers.

## Nutrition by Trimester

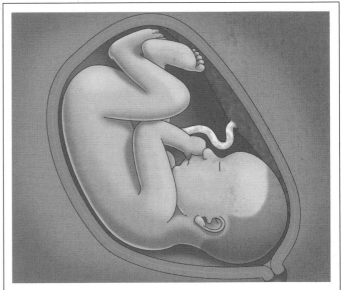

- Your iron stores can become depleted easily in the third trimester, so keep up your supply of iron-rich foods in your diet. Calcium is needed since your baby's bones and permanent teeth are continuing to develop.

- One of the building blocks for new cells is protein so include 60 grams of protein in your daily diet.

- If your weight gain is more than it should be, make sure you do not reduce your intake of these foods but rather avoid empty calories.

3RD TRIMESTER: BABY

# THE NINTH MONTH

## Your baby's gastrointestinal system is ready to start digesting food now

You are finally in your last month of pregnancy! Your baby can gain as much as half a pound each week until he is born. Some of the physical changes that happen at nine months include the development of his entire gastrointestinal system. He has a strong sucking reflex and he even makes enough enzymes to be able to digest food. The fine body hair and cheesy coating that protected his skin will begin to disappear this month so that by the time he is born, very little lanugo or vernix remains.

Reproductive changes are happening, too. If you are expecting a boy, his testicles will be fully descended during this month. For a girl, her labia will also be developed by now.

### Highlights at Nine Months

- baby gains about half a pound per week
- gastrointestinal system complete
- lanugo and vernix begin to disappear
- lifts and moves head
- testicles descend fully
- labia fully developed
- able to communicate with cries

*Digestion*

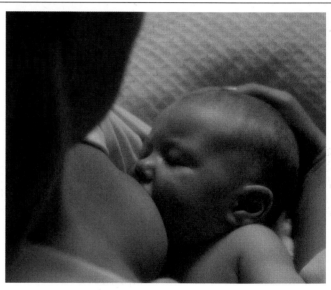

- Your baby will already have a supply of digestive enzymes that are in place in the last month before she is born.

- These enzymes help her digest food when she begins to drink breast milk or formula.

- They are crucial in helping her to break down various types of food groups in order for her body to use the nutrients.

- Additional digestive enzymes are found in breast milk which help baby digest food more readily.

During the last month, your baby is making huge leaps in her motor abilities. It may surprise you to know that your baby can lift and move her head right away after she is born. Your baby now has the ability to alert you with her cries when she is hungry, overstimulated, or uncomfortable. The good news is that it doesn't take you long to learn your baby's different cries and how best to respond.

**ZOOM**

By thirty-seven weeks of pregnancy, you will no longer be considered preterm. If your baby decides to arrive a few weeks earlier than expected, most care providers would not try to stop your labor from happening. The good news is that most babies are developed enough in terms of their digestion and respiration that they do quite well even if they are a couple of weeks ahead of schedule.

## Newborns Look Like . . .

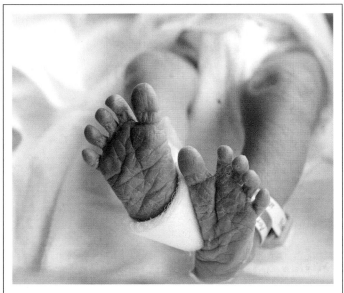

- Let's face it: Babies are very cute around six months of age.

- But right after they are born, they usually look more like your grandfather.

- Their skin looks red, wrinkled, and blotchy. They have extra hair on their face but not much on their heads.

- No matter what they look like, within a few days after they are born, you will fall madly in love!

## Baby Talk

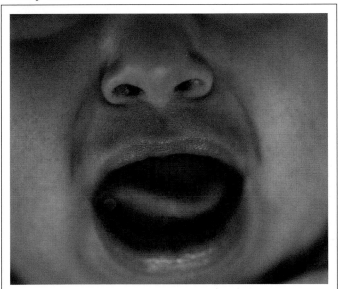

- Babies talk to us from the first moments of life.

- Even though you might try to shush your baby's cries, this is his primary means of communicating.

- Within a few days, you will be able to tell when he is hungry, cold, wet, overstimulated, in pain, or simply needing to be close to you.

- When your baby cries, it is a great idea to run through possible ways to help him as you are getting to know one another.

# PREPARING YOUR BODY

## Techniques for preparing your pelvic floor muscles for labor include Kegel exercises and perineal massage

Giving birth to your baby is one of the most physically demanding events of your life. You wouldn't dream of running a marathon without preparing your body, so why not get ready for birth with the same dedicated training?

Kegel exercises are a way to strengthen the muscles in your pelvic floor. Kegels are also helpful in preparation for labor and birth in a number of ways. As you become more familiar with when your pelvic floor muscles are relaxed, you will be able to relax, or "bulge," your pelvic floor more easily during pushing. Another way Kegel exercises help is in recovery from childbirth. If you practice Kegel exercises throughout your postpartum period, it brings greater blood flow to your

### Benefits of Kegel Exercise

- strengthens pelvic floor
- helps identify relaxed/tense muscles
- assists in recovery
- reduces bladder leakage

*How to Kegel*

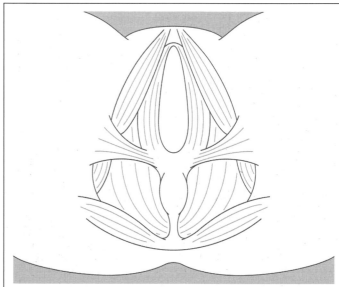

- You can find these muscles by stopping the flow of urine when you are using the bathroom.

- Tighten these muscles gradually and then hold them for a count of five, then gradually release.

- Continue practicing Kegel exercises throughout the day, even while you are at work (not when you are urinating).

- Practice sets of ten to twenty Kegels per day.

pelvic floor to increase healing if you had stitches or any tearing. Kegels are also a great way to keep your pelvic floor strengthened and toned to reduce leakage of urine during and after pregnancy and later in life.

Perineal massage helps to soften and increase the flexibility of the skin and connective tissue between your vagina and rectum. It can be done by the mother or her sexual partner. Research shows that first-time mothers who started perineal massage at thirty-four weeks and performed it daily increased their chances of not tearing at all during birth.

## Perineal Massage

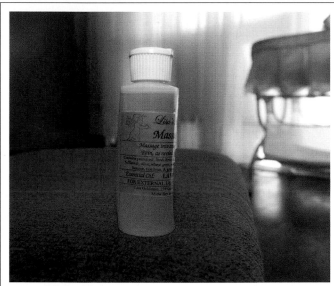

- You might feel reluctant or skeptical of doing perineal massage at first.

- Unless you have an infection or other health issues, perineal massage can only be a benefit to you.

- You might find it helpful to use a water-based lubricant, such as K-Y gel.

- Moms could also use vitamin E oil, pure vegetable oil, or olive oil if preferred. (Do not use baby oil or mineral oil.)

### How to Do Perineal Massage

- Wash your hands.

- Stand in the shower with one foot up or sit on the toilet. Lubricate your thumb and first two fingers with water-based lubricant or oil.

- Insert your fingers or thumb into your vagina up to the second knuckle.

- Massage in a U-shape, pressing gently.

- Also massage the tissue between your thumb and fingers. Gradually increase the amount of pressure until it burns.

- Focus on relaxing as you massage. Over time you should notice the tissue becoming softer.

- Massage five minutes daily from thirty-four weeks until you go into labor.

# PACKING YOUR LABOR BAG

## Two essentials for your labor bag are snacks for dad and personal items for mom

Expectant parents usually take everything but the kitchen sink with them for their first baby. What do you need to pack in your labor bag? One of the most forgotten items is a camera, but many cell phones now come with cameras, so that can be a lifesaver if you forget yours.

If your place of birth does not carry birth balls, be sure

you bring one from home. Other labor tools you might like include microwavable hot packs, massagers, and CDs with mom's favorite music. Also bring lip balm in case of chapped lips after all of that breathing.

You might prefer to bring your own robe to wear over your hospital gown and some slippers. Mothers might also like

### What to Pack
- birth ball
- lightweight robe
- slippers or extra socks
- extra pillows
- food and beverages for dad
- labor tools
- toiletries/cosmetics
- lip balm
- hard candies/lollipops
- Gatorade or other energy/electrolyte drinks
- plastic drink bottles with cap and straw
- breastfeeding pillow
- clothing for baby and diaper bag
- loose-fitting clothes for mom
- digital and/or disposable camera
- cell phone
- list of phone numbers
- change for vending machines

### What to Wear

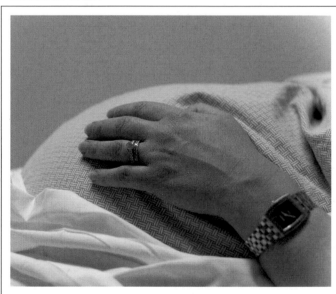

- Some mothers might prefer to wear their own nightgown or other clothes during labor.

- It is also nice to have your own robe and slippers for times when you need to step outside your room.

- Make sure that what you choose to wear in labor has easy access to your arms for starting an IV if necessary.

- Keep in mind that what you wear in labor may not be salvageable, so be sure it is not a clothing item you are attached to.

the feel of their own pillows to use after birth. Don't forget to throw in your breastfeeding pillow as well.

Snacks are essential for your birth team. Items like granola bars, crackers, fruit, and nuts are portable and do not require refrigeration. In labor mom may prefer beverages that are diluted with water. Throw some hard candies in your bag for quick energy.

For after birth, don't forget to pack clothing for your baby and loose-fitting clothes that you might have worn when you were about six months pregnant.

## Birth Balls

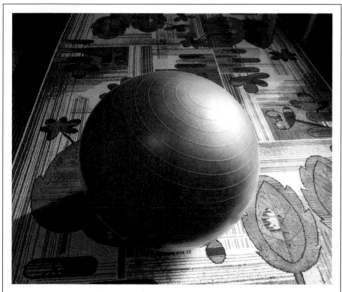

- You can bring your own ball or find out if your place of birth provides them.

- Be sure to keep the ball covered with a disposable pad or towel before you sit or lean over on it.

- Remember that you will feel less stable on your feet during labor.

- Your labor partner(s) need to support you as you sit, move around, or get up from a seated position on the ball.

## Snacks for Dad

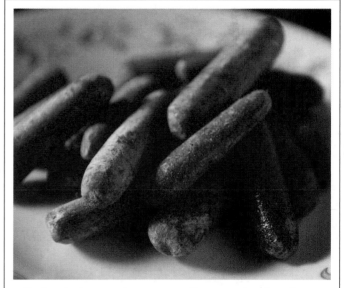

- Dad and other members of the birth team will need fuel to keep them going.

- Items such as fruit, energy or protein bars, crackers, or a sandwich are great for quick energy.

- Be aware that the odors of what you eat could be objectionable to mom, such as tuna, peanuts, coffee, or foods with garlic.

- To be safe, don't forget to throw in toothbrushes and/or gum or mints.

LABOR & BIRTH

# IDENTIFYING LABOR
## Changes in contractions over time means you are in true labor

One of the most frequently asked questions by expectant moms is, "How will I know when labor starts?" Here are some basic rules of thumb to help you identify labor.

First of all, notice if your contractions are changing over time. Are contractions lasting longer over time? Does it feel like the intensity of the contractions is increasing? When you time contractions, is the time between contractions getting closer and closer together? Do your contractions require more attention?

In addition to noticing changes in contractions, you will also want to observe any new labor symptoms that are different. Are you noticing changes in vaginal discharge? Have you seen any bright red, bloody discharge (called show)? Are you feeling pain with contractions that moves lower, for example

### Labor Signs to Notice

- Contractions are becoming closer together.

- Contractions are increasing in intensity.

- Contractions are getting longer.

- Water breaks.

- Presence of bloody show.

- Labor pain changes.

- Mom notices bodily or emotional changes.

### Timing Contractions

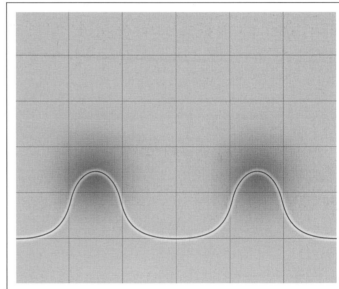

- You do not need to record every contraction during labor, only as a second check to confirm changes in labor.

- Your birth partner can time the entire length of each contraction, or the duration.

- Your partner can also monitor the time in between contractions, the interval.

- The interval is measured from the start of one contraction to the start of the next.

to your lower back? Is there any pelvic pressure with contractions or pressure in your pelvic floor from time to time? Do you notice that you feel queasy now? Labor, when it is the real thing, changes over time.

If you are getting regular contractions but they remain the same, you may be in the early, or prodromal, phase of labor, which is often characterized by contractions that do not increase in intensity. Prodromal labor can last for hours and even days, and it is a very normal aspect of labor for many mothers.

## Laboring at Home

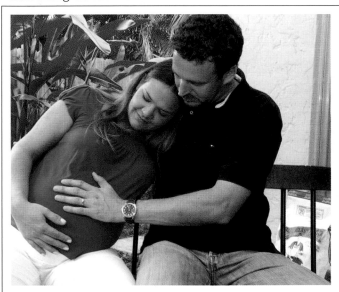

- In most cases when you have a low-risk pregnancy and you have plenty of support, you can benefit from staying at home.

- This allows you to keep yourself hydrated and eat lightly in between contractions and before labor becomes more intense.

- If contractions begin at night and are mild, try to go back to sleep to conserve energy.

- Staying at home in early labor also allows you to watch for labor changes in your own environment with privacy.

## When to Call

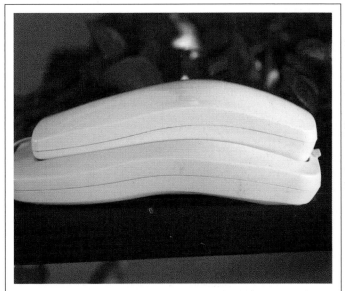

- Call your care provider if you have questions during early labor when you are at home.

- Definitely plan to contact him or her when your contractions are about three to five minutes apart, lasting for about sixty seconds for at least one hour.

- You may need to go to your place of birth sooner if you have a history of fast labors or you live far from your place of birth.

- Check with your provider ahead of time if you may have other health issues that require attention.

LABOR & BIRTH

# GRANDPARENTS' ROLE AT BIRTH

## Grandparents should be familiar with the parents' birth plan if they attend the birth of their grandchild

One of the first things to do before you make plans to include extra family members at your birth is check with your birth place. Some hospitals may limit the number of support people present in the room at any given time.

If grandparents or any other family will be participating in the birth, reading pregnancy books and attending the childbirth class are helpful ways to support the expectant couple. It is also crucial that the grandparents are knowledgeable about the mother's birth plan, so they know what her preferences are.

Don't forget that your plans may need to change. Though it may seem like a wonderful idea to include family members in your birth, it may become burdensome during labor

### Tips for Grandparents

- Attend childbirth class.
- Read pregnancy-related books.
- Become familiar with the birth plan.
- Care for older children or pets.
- Make meals and/or provide support at home.

*Labor Support from Family*

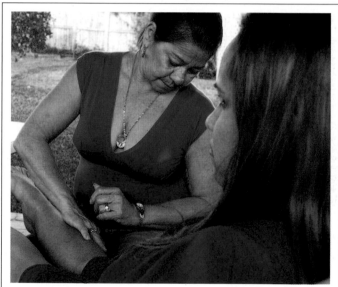

- If you plan to have relatives support you during labor, plan ahead so that they know what their role will be.

- One suggestion is to have one extra family member take childbirth classes with you to learn ways to help you during labor.

- Perhaps one family member could be in charge of taking photos or making sure mom is keeping up with her fluids.

- You might also have a family member ready to take over for when dad needs to take breaks.

when mom wants quiet and privacy. For that reason, parents should have an understanding with all family members that if the mother changes her mind about having people in the room, they will respect her wishes.

If either the grandparents or the parents are not comfortable sharing the birth event together, then perhaps grandparents can come in after the baby is born. Or they can care for older siblings or pets at home. Why not make some meals to be eaten later? New parents will need support. Grandparents are often one of the best sources of comfort and guidance.

## Postpartum Support

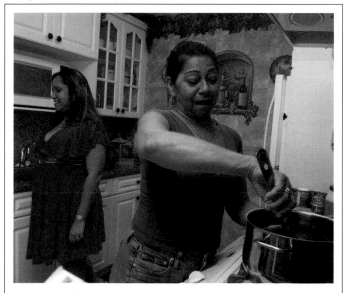

- One of the times when family support is needed the most is right after the new family gets home.

- This is often a time when moms are trying to recover, have the most questions, and have the fewest resources to help them out.

- The new mother will need nutritious meals to help her recover, so grandparents who enjoy cooking will be of great service to the new family.

- Even having an extra set of hands to give mom some much needed rest is helpful.

## Ongoing Help

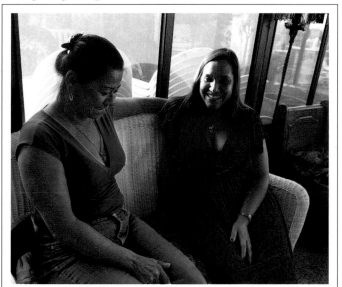

- Simply knowing that grandparents have been through the sleepless nights and daytime worries of parenting before is a comfort to the new mother and father.

- It is not uncommon for the new parents to need to connect more often with their own parents in baby's early weeks and months.

- The good news is that most grandparents today look for opportunities to help care for their children and grandchildren.

- Grandparents are often ready to offer babysitting services for new parents.

LABOR & BIRTH

# YOUR RESOURCE LIST
## Start building your list of resources now to make it easier to find information when you need it

As self-sufficient as you try to be, usually you learn fairly soon that you cannot do it all alone. Pregnancy is a time when many women begin to learn that lesson. As a new mother, you will have countless questions about what is normal and what is not. There are also times when you simply need to ask for help. Perhaps asking for help is one of the most important

lessons you learn from the childbearing years!

Having a list of resources at your fingertips so that you can get the timely help you need is going to be essential for you. The good news is that you probably don't need to start your resource list from scratch, since you may be already using many of these services. When you are listing the organizations

### Resources to Get You Started

- primary care provider (mother)
- primary care provider (baby)
- birth doula or postpartum doula
- lactation consultants
- breastfeeding warm line
- La Leche League
- chiropractors
- acupuncturists
- massage therapists
- support groups for new parents
- counselors/psychiatrists
- local faith-based groups
- pharmacy
- neighbors

### Easy Access

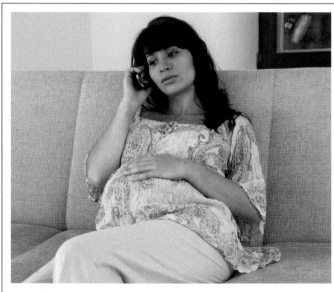

- It is not unusual for moms to feel a sense of chaos in the postpartum period.

- It can be frustrating to not have a telephone number readily available when you need it most.

- You might want to keep your list of resources handy in your phone or BlackBerry.

- Or if you prefer the old-fashioned way, have your resource list accessible in a small address book in your purse.

and professionals in your community, be sure to find out if there are "after hours" phone numbers if you need support or you have questions outside the hours of nine to five.

To make your lives simpler, especially in the chaos of the first few weeks at home, put your resource list all in one place where you won't have trouble finding it later. You may decide to put all of the contact information from your resource list right in your phone or BlackBerry.

## Home with Baby

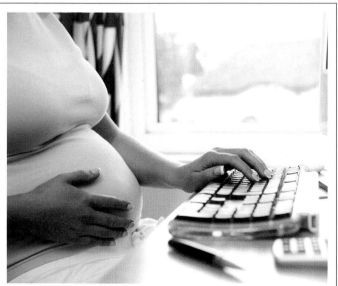

- You will undoubtedly have questions and concerns during pregnancy.

- However, often the time when moms feel the most cut off from support is when they get home after birth.

- One of the benefits of putting your resource list together now is that you do not have to be spending hours on the phone tracking down resources during the most stressful times.

- Words to the wise—your resource list may be stress prevention.

## Support Groups

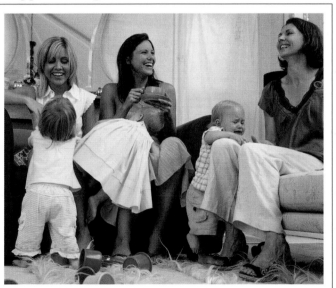

- New mothers' groups can be one of the most beneficial sources of support for moms in the early weeks or months after baby arrives.

- Your local community or faith-based groups often have information about support systems in your area for new mothers.

- A good place to start if you are breastfeeding is to contact La Leche League.

- If you have trouble finding a group, why not start your own?

LABOR & BIRTH

# LIFE AFTER BABY

## Pamper yourself in the last few weeks of pregnancy to slow down your busy pace and conserve energy

When your due date is right around the corner, one of your jobs is to finish a few last-minute projects to make your life less stressful after baby arrives. However, the first and most important thing for expectant mothers to do is to rest as much as possible. It will be a long time before you will get a full night's sleep.

The last few weeks of pregnancy are an ideal opportunity to pamper yourself. Spend a day at the spa. Even just a long, relaxing bath is great if your budget is tight. Consider shortening your work hours or stop working a few days before your due date. Take naps, read novels, drink a cup of tea, or write e-mails to people you want to connect with.

### Nesting Tips

- Pamper yourself.
- Finish little projects.
- Wash baby clothes.
- Freeze meals.
- Rest when possible.

*Energy Conservation*

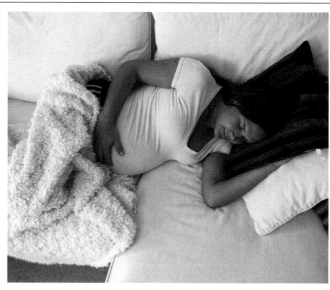

- Listen to your body and rest throughout your day when you can.

- Your body will start to tell you that you will need more and more rest in the last few weeks before labor begins.

- Moms may be tempted to induce labor because they are not sleeping at night.

- Remember that your body is now starting to prepare for sleeping in only blocks of a few hours at a time.

178

Part of your natural "nesting" does take over in the last few weeks, and that might motivate you to clean your closets at 2:00 a.m. Why not make sure your baby clothes are washed and put away during your last month of pregnancy? This will certainly save you many hours of time rather than waiting until after you bring baby home. You might want to finish any of those little projects that you have been procrastinating on, like having the leaky faucet fixed or the oil changed in your car, since it will be harder to schedule those things later.

If you are doing any cooking, why not double the recipe and put the rest in the freezer? If you are diligent about doing this in your last month, you might manage to freeze enough meals to last for two or more weeks. Just remember that your nesting urge is designed to give you energy for labor, so conserve what energy you have as much as possible.

## Treat Yourself

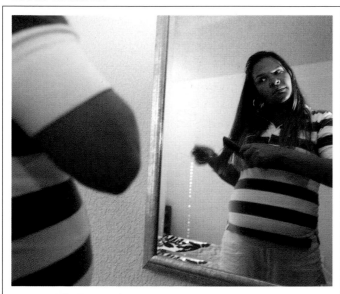

- It won't be long before your entire day revolves around your baby's needs.

- Take some time now to pamper yourself.

- Splurge on a facial, manicure, pedicure, or all three! Or enjoy a meal at your

favorite restaurant with your husband or a good friend.

- It could be a while before you do those things without needing a sitter.

## Little Projects

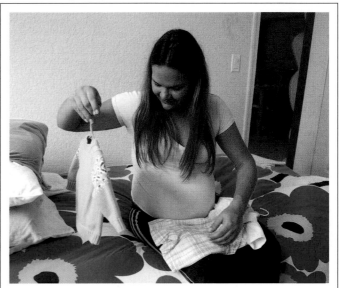

- The last few weeks of pregnancy are not the time to be starting major projects.

- Unless a project is nearing completion at this stage, don't bother starting it.

- You may just be adding to your stress to have half-

done projects around the house for weeks while your focus will need to be on your baby.

- Use this time to do little things like organize baby items in the nursery or wash and fold baby's clothing.

179

# YOUR BIRTH TEAM

## Your birth plan can be separated into sections according to the duties of each team member

Writing a birth plan provides a way to communicate your preferences prior to labor to your birth team; it's about educating yourself through reading, research, and independent, informed decisions. Birth plans are not for everyone, but for some mothers, it helps them to know that they will be included in decision making regardless of what happens.

There are a number of written birth plan formats to use. You could write a paragraph about what is most important to you. Another way is to divide your preferences according to the stage of labor where they apply. You can also separate your birth plan into sections specifically for each member of your birth team.

### Who Does What?

Obstetrician/midwife:

- breaking water, episiotomies, positions for pushing

- ordering meds, Pitocin, IV, approval for fluids/food and monitoring

Labor Nurse:

- placement of IV, IV meds, checking vital signs, monitoring baby

- newborn procedures

Anesthesiologist:

- epidural options (walking or light epidural, if available)

- approval for eating/drinking, if allowed

### Communication Tool

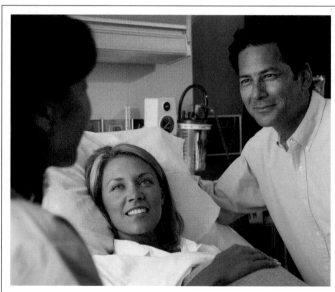

- Some parents mistakenly believe that a birth plan is writing out a list of demands for their care provider to follow.

- Birth plans should be written in conjunction with your care provider well before labor.

- If your care provider practice has several obstetricians or midwives in the group, be sure to share your birth plan with each care provider.

- When you get to your place of birth, have your birth plan accessible for the rest of the birth team.

Since your labor nurse will be responsible for starting an IV if one is used, you could write a section about your preferences regarding fluids or using a saline lock and put it under a heading for her to read. Since your obstetrician or midwife would be responsible for procedures such as breaking your water, this issue could be indicated in a section for your primary provider in your birth plan. Knowing the policies in your chosen place of birth will also help you to keep your expectations realistic.

· · · · · · · · · · · · YELLOW ● LIGHT · · · · · · · · · · · ·

A note about the labor nurse: Parents may not realize that, at most hospitals, labor nurses are very busy and sometimes attend to more than one patient at a time. Research indicates that nurses spend only about 10 percent of their time doing supportive, bedside care to the mother (i.e., the type of care doulas provide). While a labor nurse can help you periodically, be sure you have additional forms of support, such as your partner, family members, or a birth doula.

## About You

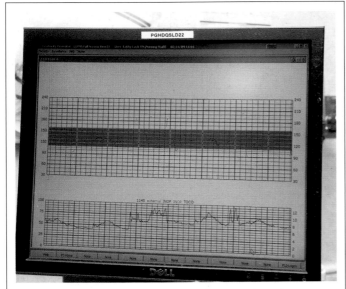

- Your birth plan is very specific to your needs and preferences during and immediately after your birth.

- Some parents include an introductory paragraph that describes a little about them.

- It is not a good idea to copy another person's birth plan or use a checklist off the Internet, since your needs will be different. A good place to start is choosing three to four issues that are the most important to you.

## Special Needs

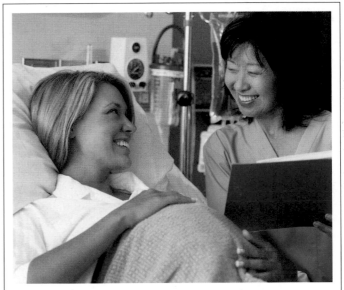

- The birth plan is an excellent place to indicate special needs of the mother or family.

- These could include special diets or any specific cultural or religious preferences.

- Mothers who have had a previously difficult birth, a negative experience in a medical setting, or a past history of abuse may choose to disclose that in a birth plan.

- Allergies to foods, medications, or other medical substances can also be added to your plan.

# PAIN MEDICATIONS

## Mothers can benefit from waiting until labor is progressing well before choosing an epidural for pain relief

The significant majority of mothers in the U.S. today choose to use an epidural during their labors. Epidurals are typically given by the anesthesiologist when a mother is in the active phase of labor. There are some benefits to waiting until your labor is progressing well before getting an epidural. If you get an epidural when your cervix is well-dilated and your baby has rotated and moved down into your pelvis, it will be less likely to slow labor.

If you are interested in having a lighter pain block during labor, you might request a "light" epidural. Another option that mothers might consider is a "walking" epidural that allows them the possibility of walking to the bathroom.

### Pros of Epidurals

- one of the easiest ways to conserve energy
- helpful when mothers are having trouble relaxing
- effective for long labors
- useful when mothers have unresolved fear going into childbirth

### Cons of Epidurals

- mother is in bed with monitors, BP cuffs, and possibly a urinary catheter
- can slow the natural course or progress of labor
- likely to increase mother's pushing time
- can decrease the mother's blood pressure

### The Epidural Procedure

- IV fluids given to prevent mother's BP from dropping.
- Anesthesiologist numbs the area in mother's lower back with a local anesthetic.
- Needle is placed into the epidural space, which is outside of the covering of the spinal cord.
- A tiny catheter is threaded into the epidural needle and the needle is removed.
- The catheter is taped to mother's back.

When you are taking your tour, be sure to check if these epidural options are available.

Narcotics are also given by your labor nurse during active labor. Unlike an epidural, which blocks most of the sensation of pain, narcotics can relax you in between contractions, but they do not reduce labor pain. Narcotics can have unpleasant side effects, such as nausea and sedation and make it harder for you to cope with pain. Choosing any type of pain medication is a big decision, so you will need to be fully informed about the pros and cons before you know what is best for you.

**ZOOM**

While not all experts agree, recent studies show that mothers who receive epidurals prior to active labor had a two-fold increase in their chances of having a cesarean. Here is another reason to wait until you are in active labor before getting an epidural.

## IV Narcotics

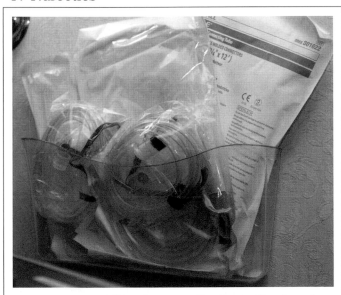

- Narcotics work differently than regional anesthesia like an epidural, since they do not numb the pain.

- The nurse gradually administers the narcotic into your IV and the medication travels throughout your bloodstream.

- The sleepy effect from the medications will usually last about one to two hours.

- If you have had reactions to any medication in the narcotic family such as Demerol, morphine, or OxyContin, let your care provider know.

## Making the Decision

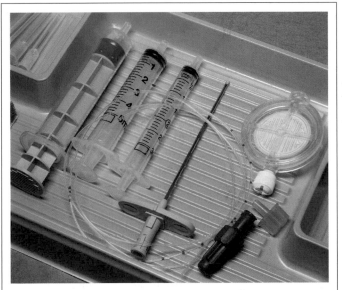

- Every woman who gives birth is confronted with the decision about pain medication.

- Knowing that you have several options to choose from can make the idea of labor pain less frightening.

- Many women choose pain medication, while others decide to go medication-free.

- However, there is no right or wrong decision; the best decision is the one that suits your needs as the laboring woman.

# LABOR POSITIONS

## A favorite labor position is for mother to stand and lean on her partner during contractions

Having positioning strategies is important to a successful labor. Many mothers find that the labor bed makes contraction pain even worse and that staying upright or walking in between contractions provides some relief. If you can to move about freely during labor, it will be more comfortable. It is one of the best ways to keep your labor moving.

One of the most effective positions to turn a baby's head is lunging. Since back pain is common, using a hands-and-knees position can help take some of the baby's weight off your back. Leaning over (hugging) the birth ball or the top of the labor bed while kneeling is even better, since you don't have to hold yourself up. Sitting on the ball when you get

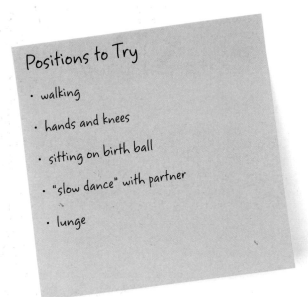

Positions to Try

• walking

• hands and knees

• sitting on birth ball

• "slow dance" with partner

• lunge

*Slow Dance*

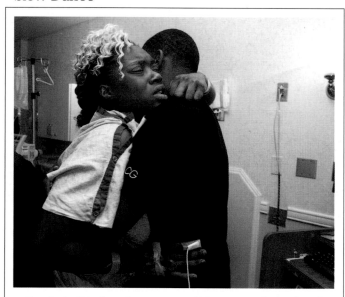

- Gravity in this slow dance position is great to help your baby move down into your pelvis.

- Dad can help support mom so that she doesn't have to hold herself up.

- Using some of your favorite relaxing music is a good distraction from the contraction pain.

- Swaying your hips in rhythm to the music can help a baby rotate to get into an anterior position in your pelvis.

tired often feels better than sitting on the bed or a chair. Partners can be wonderful support to the laboring mother and hold her in a "slow dance" position during and in between contractions.

Remember that combining other comfort techniques with positioning will be more effective for pain relief. For example, hands and knees with back pressure or a hot pack on the lower back is much more effective than the position alone.

## MAKE IT EASY

Laboring in bed: When mobility is limited, think creatively! Bring out the music. Use massage oils or lotions. Change positions in the bed as often as possible. Use a warm rice sock if mom is chilled or some cool cloths if she is hot. Dim the lights if she likes that or open the blinds to enjoy the sun during the day. Offer her ice chips or clear fluids if possible.

### Lunge

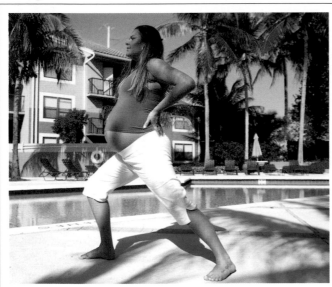

- Lunging is one of the most effective positions to turn baby's head to face your back.

- Mom should place one leg up on the seat of a chair that is pushed up against a wall.

- During contractions, she lunges back and forth toward her bent knee.

- It may take as many as five contractions to move your baby's head, so stick with it! This position can be performed in bed if needed.

### Kneeling

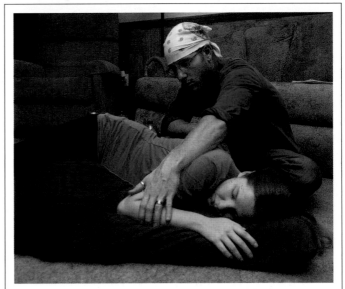

- This position can be used with any normal hospital bed, as the head can be raised as high as is comfortable for mom.

- Taking the baby's weight off of mom's back in this position can help to relieve back labor.

- Use a pillow to cushion the top of the bed and have mom drape over the top.

- Her birth partners can use massage or place cold or hot packs to her back easily in this position.

# BIRTH PLAN OPTIONS

## Discussing your preferences for a birth position should be included in your birth plan

There are many additional options to consider adding to your birth plan. Perhaps you would prefer to drink fluids but would be okay with a saline or heparin lock. This lock allows your nurse to quickly have access to a vein in the case of a complication. You might think about how you feel about having your water broken, or episiotomies. If your labor slows

down a bit, you may decide that you are okay with Pitocin being used. If you prefer natural methods to stimulate labor, be sure someone in your birth team is knowledgeable about using them.

What about options with regard to fetal monitoring? If you are not receiving pain medication, you should have the option

Labor Options to Include:

- eating/drinking

- IV fluids/saline lock

- monitoring preferences

- use of Pitocin/other methods

- positions for labor

- episiotomy/other methods

- breaking of water; timing and preferences

- positions for pushing and birth

### Avoiding Tears

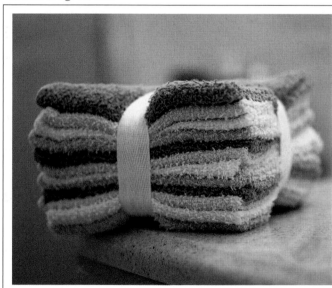

- Some care providers may use a warm compress or perineal massage to help the tissues of your perineum stretch.

- Another helpful technique to help your body stretch naturally is to slow the birth of the head.

- Your care provider may instruct you to push very slowly when your baby's head is being born.

- Research shows that when the care provider assists mother in slowing the birth this way, large tears are minimized.

(at some institutions) to have your baby monitored intermittently or checked by hand with a Doppler. Some birth settings have portable monitors (known as telemetry), where you can walk around your room or out into the labor and delivery floor while radio waves pick up your baby's heart beat.

Remember that your birth plan is not a list of dos and don'ts for your birth team, but rather a communication tool to share what is most important to you when options are available. Birth plans should remain flexible since labor is unpredictable.

**ZOOM**

Breaking water does not speed up labor: The *Cochrane Review* in 2007 compiled results from fourteen studies to see the effect of the care provider breaking the water versus not breaking it. The length of the first stage of labor remained the same. Researchers recommended that breaking your water should not be a routine part of a mother's care.

## Labor Stimulation

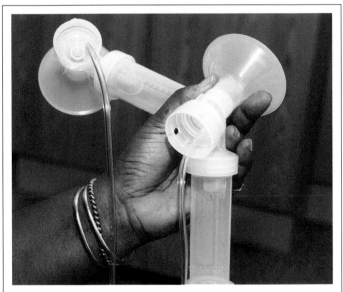

- Using the hormone Pitocin is one way to increase the strength of your contractions.

- You can also help your labor progress by walking or using position changes.

- Some mothers may find that the use of acupressure points can stimulate contractions.

- Using a breast pump or doing nipple stimulation helps to increase your body's own production of oxytocin. Use under the supervision of your care provider.

## Monitoring Baby

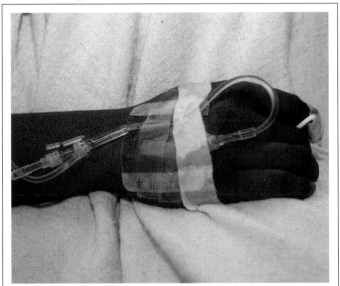

- No matter where you choose to give birth, your care provider will want to check on your baby's heartbeat frequently in labor.

- Fetal monitors include portable models that allow you the most freedom to move about.

- Most hospitals use external monitors that are strapped to your abdomen and record the baby's heart rate and contractions.

- Sometimes labor complications might require the use of an internal monitor that attaches directly to your baby's scalp.

# BABY CARE OPTIONS
## Babies are typically ready to nurse within the first thirty minutes after birth

The first hour or two after your baby is born is an ideal time to get breastfeeding off to a good start and to bond with your baby. Unless your baby needs assistance during that time from hospital staff, some parents opt to delay routine procedures. Others prefer to have procedures finished so that they can enjoy the rest of the bonding time without interruption.

Even before you are aware of any testing, your baby will have her first Apgar test at one minute and five minutes after birth. This is often done with your baby right on your chest. The nurse will look at your baby's heart rate, respiration, reflexes, muscle tone, and color for a perfect score of ten. Keep in mind that some discoloration of the feet and

**Baby Care Options**

- skin-to-skin contact
- breastfeeding
- delay newborn procedures for bonding
- no pacifiers or formula if breastfeeding
- baby bath and timing
- circumcision

*Skin-to-Skin*

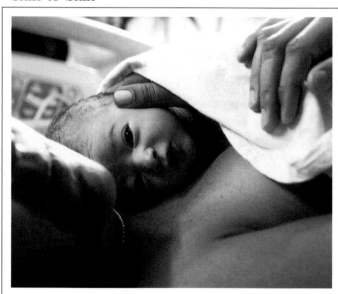

- You may want to request that your baby be placed directly on your chest after birth.

- Move any clothing so that baby's body is directly on your skin.

- Your nurse or care provider will then cover you both with a warm towel or blanket.

- This is not only a wonderful way to start bonding, but the perfect way to keep your baby warm.

hands is normal and to be expected, so a score of eight or nine is perfectly normal.

Frequently, the next thing your labor nurse will do is put antibiotic drops (erythromycin) in your baby's eyes to prevent infection. Your nurse will also be giving your baby a vitamin K shot to stimulate her blood to clot. Parents often wait anxiously to hear about their baby's birth weight and length. The baby bath and procedures like circumcision are typically done the following day, to give you and your baby time to get adjusted.

**ZOOM**

Circumcision controversy: Fewer parents in the U.S. (50 percent) are opting to do circumcision today compared to fifty years ago (80 percent). More parents who opt for circumcision do it for cultural or religious reasons, rather than health benefits. The American Academy of Pediatrics says that there is not enough current evidence to recommend routine circumcision.

## Baby's Weight

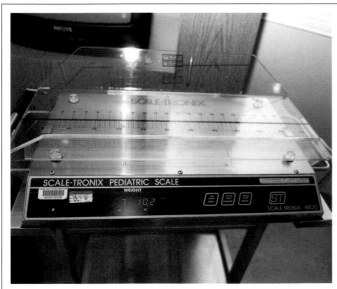

- You can request that your baby be weighed and measured after you have had an opportunity to breastfeed.

- Don't be surprised to see that your baby will lose weight in the first few days.

- It is normal for babies to initially lose about 10 percent of their birth weight.

- By two weeks of age, most babies are right back on track and have reached their birth weight again.

## Antibiotic Ointment

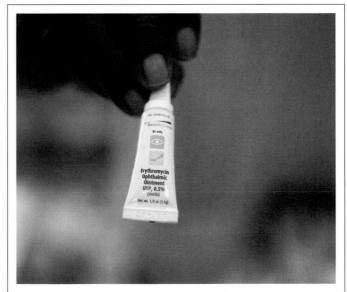

- Your nurse will be putting antibiotic eye ointment in your baby's eyes, usually within the first hour after birth.

- This ointment typically is erythromycin.

- This is a routine treatment to help prevent eye infec-

tion if the mother has an STD such as chlamydia.

- Some parents prefer to wait until they have had a chance to hold or breastfeed their baby before the baby's eyes are treated. Delaying the treatment for an hour or so after birth does not diminish its efficacy.

# UNEXPECTED SITUATIONS

## Your birth plan should include unexpected situations such as a cesarean or a baby in the NICU

An excellent reason to keep your birth plan flexible is due to unforeseen circumstances regarding you or your baby's health over which you have no control. Even though parents may plan for a homebirth, it is possible that they might eventually have a cesarean. A mother might also plan to go into labor on her own, only to realize that an induction is necessary because her blood pressure goes up in the last week. These are all difficult adjustments to make, but knowing that you have options and decisions even in the unexpected circumstances can be a help to parents.

One of the most troubling outcomes for parents can be if your baby is admitted to the NICU (neonatal intensive care

### Coping with Changes

- Include unexpected outcomes in birth plan.

- Realize that you did not "fail."

- Explore what options you still have.

- Ask for physical or emotional support when needed.

- Recognize that grief is likely to happen.

*Operating Room*

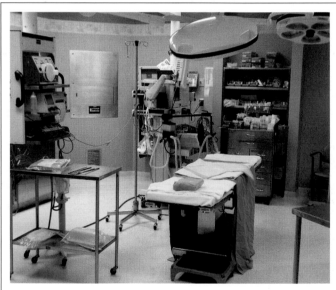

- Having a cesarean is major surgery and cannot be compared to having a vaginal birth.

- While some mothers may not have any negative feelings about having a cesarean, others will be devastated.

- Mothers who realize that their fears are becoming reality will need to grieve.

- Birth partners and family need to remember that this is a loss and respect that process for her.

unit). This can happen for any number of reasons including a baby who is preterm, a baby who is having trouble breathing, or a baby who might have an infection. Being separated from your baby like this can add to potential breastfeeding problems or cause you to feel less confident in your role as a mother. This is one of those times when asking for help when you need it will be essential. Knowing that you have an essential role in decision making can give you a sense of empowerment.

Remember that any time your labor is not what you expected or your baby has complications, grief is inevitable. Switching gears too quickly to move past your hurt only delays the grief. If you need to talk and process through your experience with a friend or counselor, don't hesitate to get the help you need.

## Separation from Baby

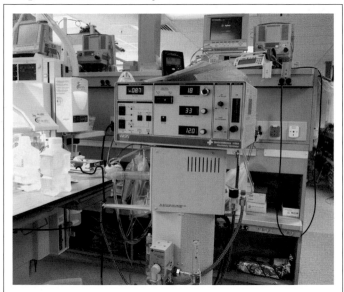

- For years, mothers were routinely separated from their babies.

- We now know that separation of mother and baby should only occur if there is a medical indication.

- Yet if that baby is yours and even if there is a medical reason, it is still not easy.

- Parents who are separated from their babies for any reason will need their questions answered and to have access to their babies as much as possible.

## Grief and Loss

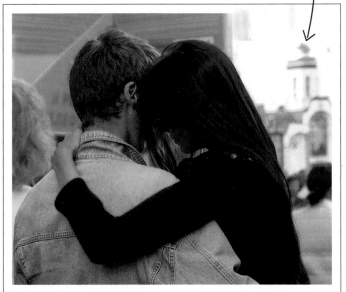

- There are many losses that parents can experience during pregnancy and labor.

- Tragedies such as miscarriage, stillbirth, and infant loss are usually at the top of the list of biggest fears during pregnancy.

- How each parent experiences grief will depend on many factors such as the parent's own life experiences and how he or she interprets this loss.

- It is critical to realize that each person will have his or her own coping mechanism to deal with grief.

# MAKING DECISIONS

## Breast milk substitutes come in handy when the supply of breast milk is not adequate

Most mothers begin to think about how they plan to feed their babies during pregnancy. If you are planning to breastfeed, you should make your decision well in advance of the birth, since it is harder to switch to breastfeeding after your baby has been formula-fed for several days.

The main reasons to breastfeed your baby are the health benefits for you and your baby. Breast milk is made specifically for humans and it includes over one hundred ingredients that are not found in infant formula. Breastfeeding has an advantage in antibodies and in bonding over bottle-feeding. However, working mothers can find breastfeeding (including locating places to pump and store breast milk at work)

### Pros of Breastfeeding

• best health benefits for mom and baby

• fewer digestive problems

• antibodies provide protection from illness

• hormones promote bonding

*Breastfeeding*

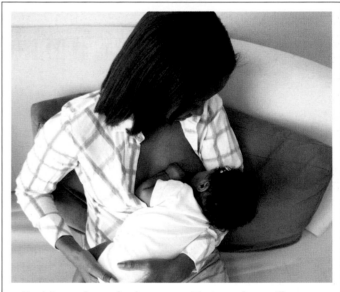

- Deciding to breastfeed your baby, even if just for a few months, is what most mothers today choose.

- Babies and mothers, with very few exceptions, enjoy significant health benefits from breastfeeding.

- Many mothers will even decide to continue breast-feeding after they return to work.

- Even though it may seem like a completely natural process, the more you know about the pitfalls, the better.

complicated. It is not uncommon for a mother who is a survivor of sexual abuse to be reluctant to breastfeed her baby and to prefer bottle-feeding, to avoid pain from her past.

Formula feeding can give the mother longer breaks in between feedings, since formula-fed babies often feel fuller. Other support people can also share in the feeding, and it is more acceptable in some regions to feed your baby formula in public than it is to breastfeed. Breast milk substitutes are convenient if the mother is unable to breastfeed or does not make enough breast milk.

**ZOOM**

How many mothers breastfeed? In 2004, according to Child Trends DataBank, the total number of mothers who breastfed their babies at all was 70 percent. At six months of age about 36 percent of mothers were breastfeeding, and by one year, 18 percent of mothers were still breastfeeding.

## Formula Feeding

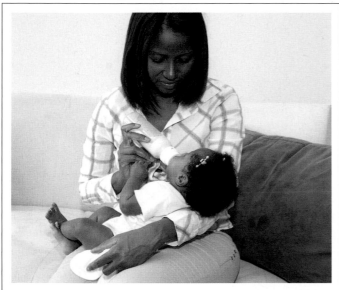

- The decision of how to feed your baby is a complicated one.

- Many working mothers lean toward feeding their babies infant formula if they are planning to go right back to work or after breast surgery.

- Others may be swayed into formula feeding for other reasons. Regardless of what decision you make, the most important issue is that you are feeding your baby lovingly and safely.

**Pros of Formula feeding**
- allows others to feed baby
- potentially longer breaks between feedings
- more culturally acceptable in public
- helpful as a supplement to breast milk

# BONDING

## Mothers and fathers can bond with their baby regardless of the method of feeding they choose

Maximizing your time of closeness and intimacy with your little one will help you grow stronger bonds with her, whether you feed your baby from your breast or give her formula in a bottle.

If you are feeding your baby from a bottle, hold her close against you. Look into her eyes and talk to her during the feeding. Stroke her soft skin, tell her how amazing she is and how much you love her! Try not to pass the baby around, but save feedings for mother and father bonding time with your baby.

Breastfeeding requires that the baby is held closely against the mother's body, whether the baby is in a football or cradle

### Bonding and Hormones

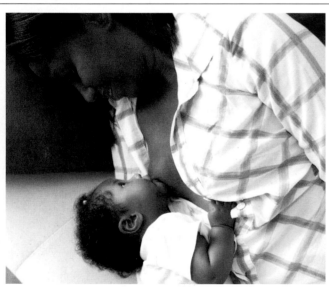

- Breastfeeding provides the optimal experience for mother-baby bonding.

- The mother will have a relaxing and sleepy sensation during breastfeeding as a result of the increased oxytocin levels.

- The baby also receives several of the mother's hormones through breast milk, including oxytocin, prostaglandins, prolactin, and thyroid stimulating hormone.

- None of these hormones are present in infant formula.

### Fathers and Bonding

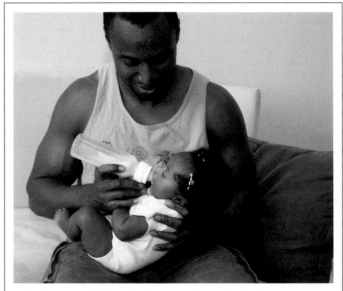

- Dads can participate in the bonding process by burping the baby at breaks in feeding.

- When mom needs a break from breastfeeding, dad can feed baby pumped breast milk.

- If you have chosen to formula-feed your baby, cuddle him close to you to promote bonding.

- Do not prop the bottle or pass the baby around for feedings, but rather save that as special bonding time for parents.

hold or the mother is lying down. The let-down of breast milk initiates the secretion of oxytocin in the mother's body, which can make the mother feel warm and very relaxed. Other ways of growing a bond with your baby include diapering, bathing, rocking, or lying next to each other. Fathers can bond with their babies by offering to give mom a break and comforting the baby as often as possible. It won't be long before you can find other ways to bond with baby. Bedtime is an ideal bonding opportunity and can include reading stories or poems or singing songs together.

*Baby Bath*

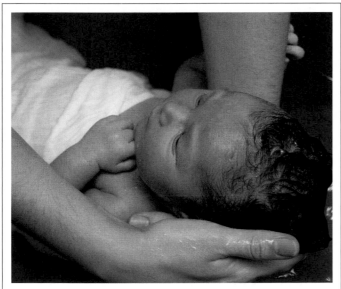

- In the pre-crawling months, your baby typically does not need a daily bath.

- Not to mention, they seldom enjoy it at first because being unclothed is just too cold.

- After a few months, however, bathing can become a fun way to spend time with your infant.

- Sometimes fathers may enjoy this time even more than mothers as part of their own bonding ritual with their infant.

Ways to Bond
- holding close during feedings
- talking to baby
- snuggling up close
- diapering
- bathing
- rocking
- singing songs
- reading stories or poems

195

# INITIATING BREASTFEEDING

## An ideal time to start to nurse your baby is within the first hour after birth

Babies are born with a strong sucking reflex and you may be surprised that they are very interested in breastfeeding in their first hour after birth. When you start to see the baby mouthing his fingers, sticking out his tongue, or rooting (when baby opens his mouth and turns his head toward you), you can be sure your baby is ready.

Start by placing your baby skin-to-skin on your chest and keep him as calm as possible. Eventually you may notice that he starts to scoot down to your breast all on his own. Hold your breast for him and keep your other hand securely around his back and buttocks.

Do not hold or press onto his head. Look for his mouth to

### Tips for Getting Started

- Start breastfeeding in the first hour.
- Look for signs baby is ready.
- Hold baby skin-to-skin on your chest.
- Keep baby calm.
- Allow baby to find breast.
- Make sure baby's mouth opens wide.
- Support breast with one hand.
- Hold baby's buttocks with other.
- Make sure baby's chin is buried into your breast.
- Check comfort.
- If latch is painful, start over.

### Keeping Baby Calm

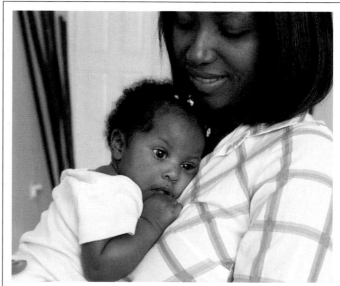

- Breastfeeding experts are realizing that babies often do better to self-attach than if we try to help them too much.

- Shoving your nipple into her mouth or pressing her head into your breast can lead to a painful latch.

- Hold your baby upright on your chest and soothe her until she is calm.

- It is best to have your breast exposed so that she can find your breast herself.

open wide and when he latches, make sure that his chin is buried into your chest with his nose not touching the breast. This helps to keep your nipple up toward the roof of his mouth.

If breastfeeding initially feels uncomfortable but after he latches it feels like a deep pressure, it is likely a good latch. If it hurts or pinches, place your finger on the side of your baby's mouth and in between the gums to break the suction and start over.

Continue to feed your baby as often as possible in the first days to encourage your breast milk to come in.

················· GREEN ● LIGHT ·············
Colostrum—Quality but Not Quantity
The first several days after birth, your baby is getting tiny amounts of colostrum at each feeding, which is perfect for your baby's small digestive system. Colostrum is higher in protein and has less sugar and fat than true breast milk. It has a laxative component to help your baby pass meconium. Last, but not least, it is plentiful in antibodies and fosters the growth of good bacteria, which fights illness.

## Open Wide

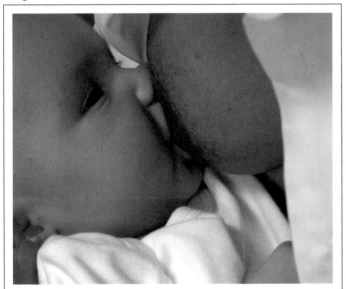

- Your baby should be opening her mouth very wide to get a good latch.

- If she nurses only on your nipple, it can lead to painful, sore, or cracked nipples.

- She will also not be able to help release more of your breast milk.

- Be patient during breastfeeding and wait for her to open wide before you offer the breast.

## A Good Latch

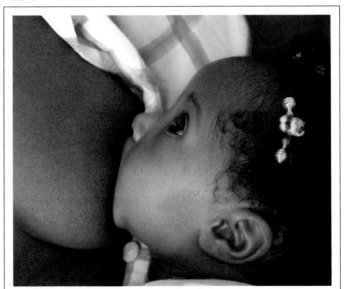

- An asymmetrical latch is best, where her lower lip covers more of the areola (the dark part of the nipple) than the upper lip.

- If the baby is positioned correctly, her chin should be pressed against the breast so that there is space between her nose and your breast.

- This asymmetrical latch helps her lower jaw get under the milk sinuses to draw the most milk from your breast.

- An asymmetrical latch is also typically more comfortable for most mothers.

197

# BREASTFEEDING TIPS

## Introducing a bottle or pacifier too soon can cause babies to become confused with breastfeeding

In the first few days after birth, it is a good rule of thumb to breastfeed whenever your baby is awake and fussy. Nursing frequently helps your milk to come in sooner and gives you and your baby more time to practice. The consistency of the breast milk changes throughout the feeding so that at the end of feeding, the milk has a higher fat content (called "hind milk"). This hind milk can help your baby gain weight, so if you try to limit the time on each breast, you could be making it harder for your baby to gain weight.

The baby, not the clock, is your best gauge for feeding schedules. Newborns can hold about 1 to 2 ounces of milk in their tummies at a time. Breast milk digests easily and quickly,

### Tips for Success

- Nurse baby frequently.

- Nurse as long as possible on the first breast.

- Watch the baby and not the clock.

- Count six to eight wet diapers per day in the first week.

- Avoid a bottle or pacifier until breast-feeding is well established.

### Hunger Cues

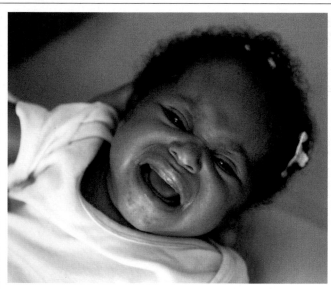

- Crying is one of the last signs of hunger a baby communicates to you.

- You should be watching for other hunger cues such as rooting or sucking on his/her fist.

- It is better to watch your baby's cues rather than pay attention to a clock for a feeding schedule.

- If you need some guidelines for feeding times, plan to breastfeed at least once every two hours throughout the day.

which is different than how your baby digests formula. Formula develops curds in the baby's stomach, making the baby feel fuller. This might mean that your breastfed newborn may be interested in eating again after only an hour.

Almost every new mother worries that her breastfed baby may not be getting enough. The number of wet diapers for the first week should be close to the number of days old your baby is. Your baby should also be having frequent dirty diapers each day. So if your baby has four wet diapers and one or more dirty diaper at four days old, she is on track! Listen for frequent swallowing during feedings and notice if your baby seems content after feedings.

Introducing a bottle or pacifier can confuse babies since they require a different sucking technique. Before you introduce a bottle or a pacifier, your baby needs to be latching well and your supply of breast milk should be plentiful.

## Getting Enough

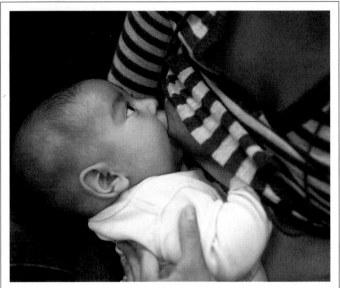

- To make sure your baby is getting enough, check for frequent swallowing during feedings.

- Does your baby seem satisfied after feedings or fall asleep after a good feeding?

- Can you count six to eight wet diapers and regular dirty diapers by one week of age?

- Mothers can also tell that their milk is letting down when they feel a tingly sensation and notice that breast milk is flowing from the opposite breast.

## Soreness

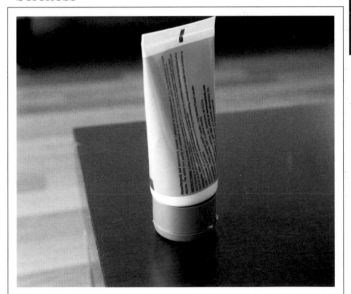

- Differentiating between normal tenderness and soreness caused by improper latching can be challenging.

- It is normal to feel a bit uncomfortable when your baby first latches, but more comfortable once your milk lets down.

- If it continues to hurt throughout your feeding, try breaking the latch by placing your finger in your baby's mouth in between her gums.

- Do not hesitate to seek help from a lactation consultant if problems continue.

# HEALTH BENEFITS

## Breast milk is loaded with disease-fighting antibodies that protect your baby from illness

One of the most amazing things about breastfeeding is that new evidence is being discovered all the time about health benefits for mothers and babies. In the short-term, breast-feeding uses up the extra fat stores your body has been put-ting on just for this purpose! Even though it is not a foolproof method of birth control, breastfeedings delay ovulation for at least the first six weeks, so it can provide a natural spacing between children. Mothers have long-term health benefits if they breastfeed long-term, including lower incidences of breast, ovarian, and uterine cancer and prevention of osteo-porosis. New evidence also shows that diabetic mothers who were breastfeeding needed less insulin.

Benefits for Baby

- ideal nutrition
- lowers risk of allergies
- decreases risk of ear infections
- lowers risk of obesity
- lowers risk of diabetes
- decreases risk of infections
- increases IQ in preterm babies

*Weight Loss*

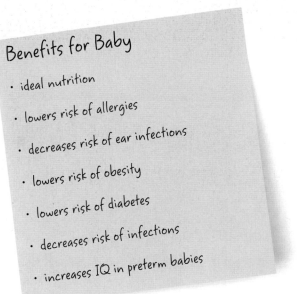

- You are likely to be more hungry and thirsty while you are breastfeeding, so make sure you get eight or more glasses of water each day. Not staying hydrated can decrease milk production.

- The good news is that breastfeeding uses up 500 or more calories a day.

- You may easily lose most of your pregnancy pounds in the first few months of breastfeeding.

- However, the timing of your post baby weight loss varies tremendously so try not to get discouraged if it takes longer than you expect.

The benefits for babies are even more impressive. Breast milk contains the perfect amount of fatty acids, lactose, water, and amino acids to help with digestion, develop his brain and help him gain weight. About 80 percent of the cells in human breast milk are "disease-fighting" cells that attack and kill viruses, bacteria, and fungi. These antibodies will lower his risk of allergies, asthma, ear infections, intestinal infections, and bronchitis. Long-term benefits include lowering the baby's risk of obesity and diabetes as well as increasing IQ among preterm babies.

## Healthier Society

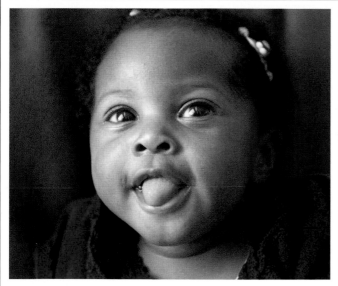

- Breastfed babies have fewer illnesses than babies that are formula-fed.

- Breastfeeding also saves on health-care costs for doctor visits, prescription medications and hospital visits.

- Breastfeeding is environmentally friendly since it reduces plastic waste from formula cans and bottle supplies. The American Academy of Pediatrics and UNICEF recommend that babies be exclusively breastfed for six months and supports breastfeeding for one full year. Nursing for up to two years is the norm in Latin America and Africa.

Health Benefits for Mom

- uses up fat stores
- delays ovulation
- lowers risk of breast cancer
- lowers risk of ovarian cancer
- lowers risk of uterine cancer
- reduces chance of osteoporosis

# RETURNING TO WORK

## Explore your work environment during your pregnancy for a clean place to pump during the day

One of the very first things you will need to do before you return to work is to purchase a good breast pump. The electric, double-pump models are popular and will typically last for several years of continuous pumping. If someone loans a pump to you, make sure you sterilize or replace the tubing and parts that come into contact with breast milk. Sterilize everything by boiling the attachments in a pot of water for twenty minutes.

Start feeding your baby pumped milk when your milk supply is well established and breastfeeding is going well, which is typically two to three weeks after birth. Do not wait until you are going back to work at six weeks to introduce a bottle,

### Checklist for Breastfeeding Moms Who Work

- Buy a double electric pump.
- Introduce bottle by around three weeks.
- Discuss pumping location with supervisor.
- Look for a clean, private location to pump breast milk.
- Research milk storage options.
- Pump and freeze milk from breast you finished on with the last feeding to build up your supply before you return to work.
- Supply day-care provider with additional formula if needed.

*Breast Pumps*

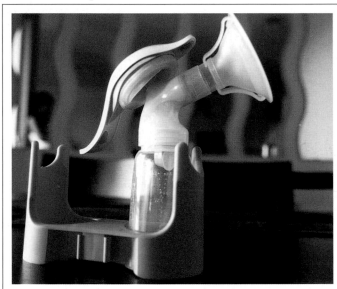

- A good electric breast pump is worth the $250-to-$350 price tag, especially since that equals the cost of about two or fewer months of formula.

- Look for one that has more suction and releases per minute, to get close to your baby's own sucking pattern.

- If you plan to pump for a shorter period of time, it may be worth renting a good pump rather than purchasing one.

- Hand-held pumps are less expensive, more portable, but less efficient to use.

since your baby is more likely to refuse it if you have waited that long.

Talk to your supervisor about the need for a place to pump. Bathrooms are not sufficient places to pump, so be on the lookout for a vacant office that is clean and private. Refrigerating breast milk is essential, so locate a place to store your milk, or store it on ice packs in a thermal bag. Pump whatever is left after feedings to store up a supply in the freezer for your baby's day-care provider. Your provider also needs a supply of infant formula in case your supply is low at times.

## Freezing and Storage

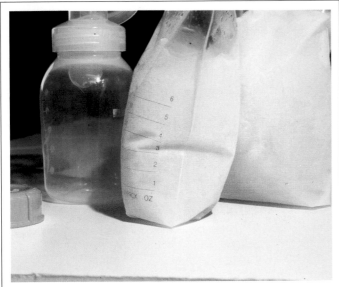

- Be sure to label all of your containers with the date before refrigerating or freezing breast milk.

- Store breast milk in small sterile bottles with screw caps or plastic lids.

- You can also find pre-sterilized nursing bags that can go right in your freezer.

- Do not save leftover milk in the bottle baby has used, since it contains bacteria. Instead, discard any milk from an unfinished bottle.

## Working and Breastfeeding

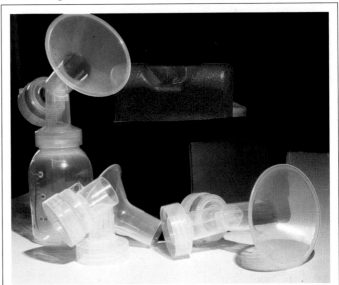

- Some mothers believe that once they go back to work, they have to stop breastfeeding.

- While it is more challenging to pump and store your milk, know that you are giving your baby the very best health benefits.

- You are also protecting your baby from illnesses she may be exposed to while in a day-care setting.

- Your body will eventually adapt to the routine of nursing both in the morning and at night when you are home.

# REALITIES OF LABOR
## One of the most common fears expectant mothers have is about labor pain

Your nine months are almost over, but labor itself is the only thing that separates you from finally meeting your baby.

For some mothers, labor is over in just a few hours. For the majority of moms, it seems labor lasts for hours and even days of contractions. The reality is that both of these labors are normal. Pacing yourself and resting when you can is ideal.

An important thing to remember is that your body will do exactly what it needs to do, and in its own time, to give birth to your baby!

The biggest fear of labor is typically the pain. How much is it really going to hurt? Well, no one can fully prepare you for the pain for a number of reasons. All women feel labor and

### Normal Labor and Planning

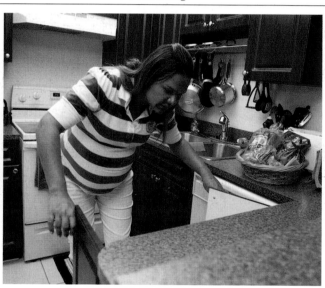

- There is no accurate definition of what is a normal labor. Normal for one woman might mean three hours and for another it might mean three days.

- Labor rarely happens in an eight-hour workday.

- Labor is difficult or even impossible to predict. It can start while you are home doing daily activities.

- Labor for each woman is unique and has its own time frame, pattern, and schedule. Don't let anyone tell you otherwise.

### Labor Is Healthy

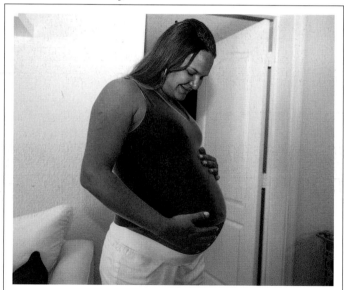

- The idea that labor is risky for mothers and babies may be one reason why some mothers are seeking scheduled cesareans.

- The truth is that spontaneous labor is healthy for your baby, since your stress hormones prepare your baby for life outside the womb.

- Research also shows that labor provides a protective benefit for future vaginal births, even if your first birth ends in a cesarean.

- There is no doubt that labor is challenging, but it is also, hands-down, the healthiest way for most women to give birth.

cope with labor pain differently. One mom might say labor was painful but she was able to cope with that pain, and another might say it was unbearable.

It is realistic to prepare for labor to hurt and hurt a lot. However, don't forget the power of your mind over the pain. Going about your everyday business and focusing on other things for as long as possible is one of the best ways of distracting yourself from the pain. Remember that it is pain with a fantastic purpose. You are only hours away from meeting your baby!

## Scheduling Labor

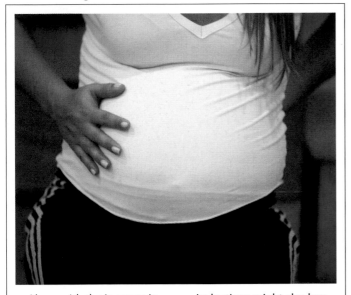

- Along with the increase in the cesarean rate, we are also seeing more and more labors being induced.

- While some of these inductions are done for definite medical reasons, others may be done for convenience.

- Inductions might also happen simply because the mother is a few days past her due date.

- Be sure you know the pluses and minuses of having your labor induced before you agree to it.

## Pain with a Purpose

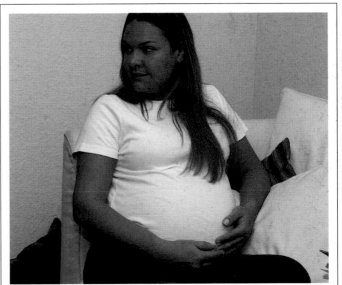

- Believe it or not, labor pain serves many purposes. It alerts you to get help when the contractions intensify.

- Pain tells you when to go to a safe place in time to have your baby.

- Pain guides you to move or change positions to help your baby move down into your pelvis.

- Labor pain also helps to tell you when you are moving ahead to a new chapter in labor, and to alert your birth team to help you in different and appropriate ways.

# COPING WITH PAIN
## Use of a tub or shower during labor can relax mothers and reduce the sensation of pain

While each mother copes with labor pain differently, there are some things that nearly all women in labor have in common. One is that they all need support in labor. Doulas, fathers, friends, and family can offer the right amount of encouragement that mothers need when they feel like giving up.

Even knowing you can "get up and do something" can help you to mentally cope with labor pain. Standing, moving around, changing positions as often as possible, and walking to the bathroom sometimes does wonders to make women feel like they have some control over an uncontrollable situation. Use of deep or patterned breathing helps a mother avoid holding her breath or hyperventilating.

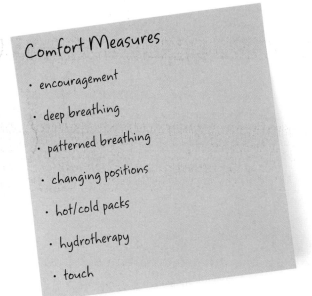

Comfort Measures

- encouragement
- deep breathing
- patterned breathing
- changing positions
- hot/cold packs
- hydrotherapy
- touch

### Heat/Cold Therapy

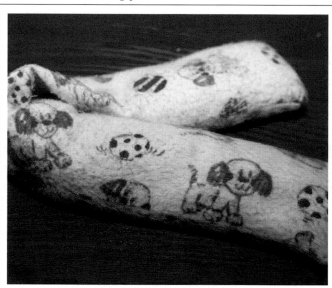

- Temperature variations can provide welcome relief to labor pain.

- Mothers may have periods of time when cold feels better than heat and vice versa.

- A cold pack that has been frozen works well for mothers who are perspiring.

- A microwaveable sock filled with rice is a convenient heat source for lower-back pain.

Techniques that actually help to block the pain sensation are things like warm or cold packs and hydrotherapy. Moms love temperature variations, so rice socks heated in the microwave for heat or frozen soda cans for cold work great! Getting into a tub lifts the baby's weight off your back and can relax you. If a tub is not available, a shower works nearly as well. Be careful to not heat the water temperature in your tub to no more than 100 degrees F.

Last, but certainly not least, is loving touch. Kneading, pressure, and stroking can ease sore muscles and comfort.

*Hydrotherapy*

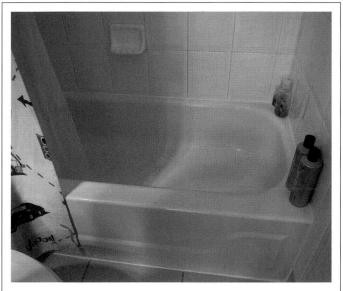

- The use of a tub or shower during labor is effective for pain relief.

- Use the removable shower head for back pain if a tub is not available at your place of birth.

- Keep the water temperature very close or just slightly higher (1-2 degrees) than your own body temperature.

- Try to avoid getting into a birthing tub too early in your labor, since it can slow contractions.

*Massage or Touch*

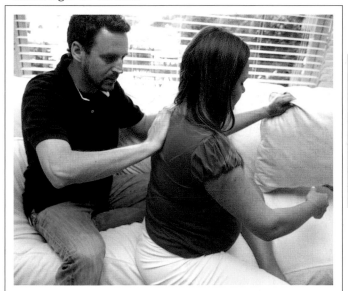

- Massage is one of the most effective techniques for comfort and relaxation.

- If birth partners massage mother's tired muscles, it can prevent soreness due to the build-up of lactic acid.

- It is important to experiment during pregnancy and early labor with various types of touch to see what mother likes and does not like.

- Keep your other techniques handy just in case mom does not want to be touched at all during labor.

# STAGES OF LABOR

## One of the most intense phases of labor for an expectant mother is transition

Labor encompasses four stages. First stage: The first stage, dilation, is made up of three phases. The early phase is when your contractions are further apart, last around thirty seconds, and are usually mild to moderate in intensity. Your cervix might be between 1 and 3 centimeters dilated. Most moms do not have as much trouble coping at this phase,

since they have a break in between contractions.

The next phase is active labor, in which your contractions are about sixty seconds long and your cervix would be dilated anywhere from 4 to 8 centimeters. Mothers need coping tools now, since the contractions are intense and harder to manage. In most cases it will be recommended that you go

Stages of Labor

The First Stage of Labor: Dilation

• early labor

• active labor

• transition

The Second Stage of Labor: Pushing

• resting

• descent

• crowning

The Third Stage: Placenta is expelled

The Fourth Stage: Recovery

*Early Labor*

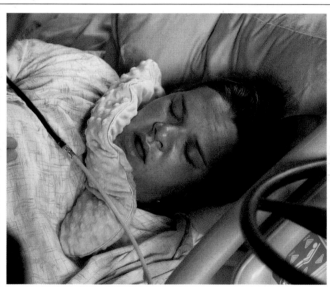

- Usually, the early phase of labor is the easiest part of labor.

- However, for many mothers, it is also the longest phase of labor.

- Unless they are being induced, most mothers will spend the early phase of their labor at home.

- Conserving your energy, resting, eating lightly, and staying hydrated are the best ways to manage early labor.

to your place of birth during active labor.

Transition is the last phase in this first stage of labor, and it is generally the most intense part of labor. The mother's cervix is about 8 to 10 centimeters dilated and she can feel pressure as her baby's head begins to press down into the cervix.

Second Stage: There are also three phases during the second stage of labor, also known as the pushing stage. Resting occurs when there is a lull between complete dilation and contractions. If there is a resting phase, mothers should wait before beginning to push, so they do not waste energy.

The descent phase occurs when mothers begin pushing during contractions. Finally, crowning is when the baby's head is low enough at the vaginal opening to remain in place in between contractions. The second stage ends with the birth of your baby.

Third Stage: Your placenta detaches from your uterus and is born any time up to thirty minutes after your baby is born.

Fourth Stage: Your uterus begins to return to its pre-pregnant size, which takes up to six weeks after your baby is born. Expect to still look about five months pregnant for a while after birth.

## Active Labor

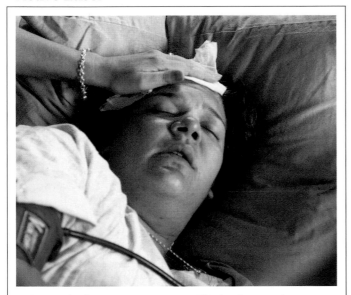

- As your body moves into active labor, contractions strengthen and become closer.

- You will need a lot of help and support from your birth team at this phase.

- This is when mothers may start to realize labor is not within their control.

- Changing positions, using deep breathing and relaxation, getting into a tub, or taking advantage of pain medication are all ways that mothers cope with active labor.

## Transition

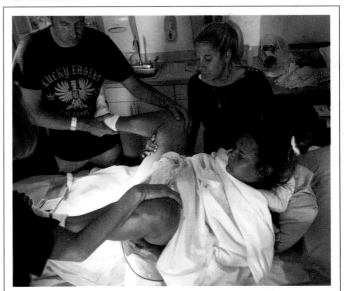

- Transition is the last phase of labor before the pushing stage begins.

- It can be the most intense and painful part of labor, but is usually one of the shortest phases.

- Your contractions may be close to two minutes long with only a minute of rest in between.

- If you are not using pain medication, you will rely heavily on the support of your birth team to cope with transition.

# SLOW VERSUS FAST LABORS

## It is much more likely you'll have a slow labor if this is your first baby

Will you have a fast and furious three-hour labor or the slow tortoise crawl that takes three days? It is very hard to predict the length of your labor. However, it is more likely for first-time mothers to take the longer route to birth their babies than it is for mothers with second or later babies. If your care provider is comfortable with it, spend as much of your long labor at home as possible. If you get to your place of birth and you are still in the early phase of labor, you may want to consider having your baby monitored for a while to be sure everything is okay and then return home. Try alternating restful activities, such as reading and napping, with more stimulating activities, such as taking long walks and making

### Coping with Slow Labors

• Stay at home as long as possible.

• Alternate between active and restful activities.

• Drink plenty of fluids.

• Eat lightly.

## Hydration

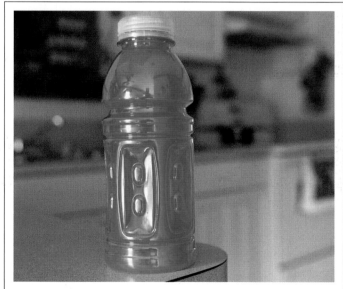

• Staying hydrated is important whether your labor is slow or fast.

• Take a sip or two of water after every few contractions to prevent dehydration.

• Drinking fluids with some sugar content will help with energy and prevent fatigue from your blood sugar dropping, if you are unable to tolerate food.

• If you are feeling nauseated, try sticking to ice chips or popsicles until the nausea subsides.

a trip to the store. One of the keys to a successful labor is to stay busy and focused doing "non-labor" activities to take your mind off contractions.

A fast labor is challenging in its own way, since your body begins intense work from the beginning. Some mothers may notice that their fast labor begins with their water breaking with one or more gushes, which are soon followed by strong contractions. Each contraction seems to strengthen from the previous one. As soon as you think you can manage the pain, the quality of the contraction changes. This makes it very hard for mothers to cope. Sometimes having a vaginal exam can be discouraging, since the intensity in the early part of labor may not line up with where she feels like she "should be" in terms of her dilation. Your birth team will play a vital role in responding to your needs, reminding you to relax and helping you stay focused during a fast labor.

## Quick Energy

- If your labor is taking many hours or even days, you will need to eat some solid food.

- Take advantage of the time you are at home to eat easily digested, low-acid foods.

- Check with your care provider and place of birth before you bring solid food to eat during labor.

- One ideal labor food is a baked white or sweet potato, since it is mild and gentle on your stomach.

*Coping with Fast Labors*

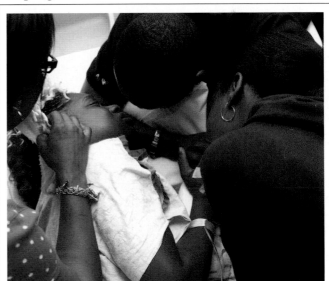

- Watch the signs of labor carefully.

- Trust your body and instincts.

- Be sure you have plenty of support.

- Communicate your needs to your birth team.

# LABOR EMOTIONS

## It is not unusual for mothers to feel "out of control" during the most intense parts of labor

Coping with labor is not just about learning the various stages and managing the physical pain. Labor brings with it a complicated mixture of emotions that can be overwhelming if parents are not prepared for the inevitable roller coaster of their feelings from one moment to the next.

When labor starts, it is not uncommon to feel both excitement ("It's finally here!") and some anxiety ("Can I do this?"). As labor intensifies, mothers emotionally become more dependent on their support team. They may express more doubts verbally or the battle may be taking place in their heads. Some mothers describe this time in labor as feeling "out of control" because their brains are incapable of their

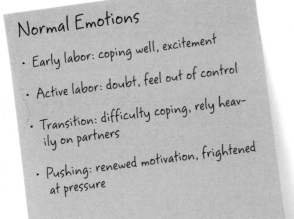

Normal Emotions

• Early labor: coping well, excitement

• Active labor: doubt, feel out of control

• Transition: difficulty coping, rely heavily on partners

• Pushing: renewed motivation, frightened at pressure

### Excitement

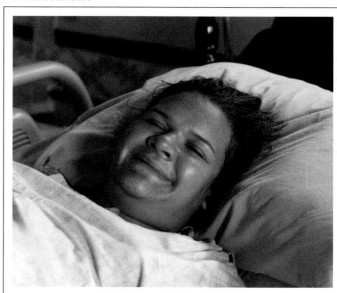

• Your baby is coming!

• Moms will often be relieved when labor finally starts.

• Early labor contractions provide ample breaks in between so mothers feel confident in their ability to handle the pain.

• Even though they know that they should be conserving energy, sometimes both parents are so excited it can be hard to rest.

normal reasoning abilities. A mother is extremely vulnerable at this time in labor, so it is crucial for her birth team to be supportive and remind her of her birth plan.

As labor progresses into the pushing stage, mothers often get a sense of renewed hope and motivation. However, mothers may wonder how they will find the energy to push, so verbal encouragement is essential. During the crowning phase, the stretching of the mother's perineum around her baby's head will cause her to feel overwhelmed once again. Reassuring her that this is normal can help mothers cope.

## MAKE IT EASY

The birth planet: One phenomenon about active labor is that high endorphin levels may cause the mom to appear to be falling asleep between contractions. She will have trouble making eye contact or conversation even when she is not contracting. This is called "going to the birth planet." Labor partners know that they should head to their place of birth when mom goes to the "birth planet."

### Coping Well

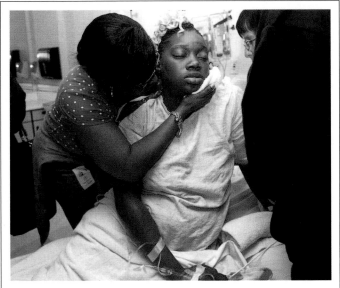

- When contractions intensify, mothers who are prepared for labor often cope well.

- Learning to "go with the flow" of labor rather than trying to control the pain is a good strategy.

- Even if moms have flickers of doubt, they manage well with plenty of support.

- One way to check if mom is coping is to observe how relaxed she is in between contractions.

### Needing Help

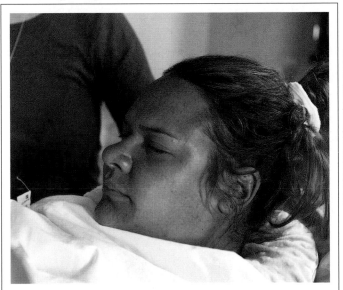

- It is not uncommon for mothers to reach a point where their coping ability changes.

- Birth partners ought to recognize that if the mother seems to "fall apart," this is a very normal labor emotion.

- Allow her to cry or express any emotion and then validate her pain and hard work.

- Be ready to jump in with several other ideas to help re-focus her energies into labor.

# PUSHING TECHNIQUES

## You can request that your epidural dosage be turned down if you are not pushing effectively

You might be thinking that pushing should be no big deal. However, there could be several things working against you. One is that epidurals reduce your sensation, so the more information you have about pushing effectively if you have an epidural, the better.

You could ask your provider to allow contractions to move

your baby's head down for as long as possible before you start to push. This is often referred to as "laboring the baby down" and it can literally save hours of pushing time. The nurse, doctor, or midwife can help by pressing her fingers toward your rectum while you push, so you know what muscles to use. A mirror is a great motivator if the nurse is able to

### Tips for Pushing

- Labor down.
- Ask nurse or caregiver to press fingers toward your rectum.
- Use a mirror to motivate you to push.
- Have the epidural turned down.
- Change positions.
- Ask for more time to push.

*Mirror*

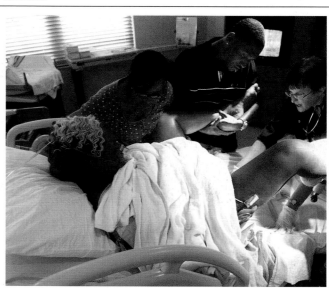

- A mirror can be an encouragement when pushing is long and slow.

- Mom may need the reassurance to know she is getting close to meeting her baby.

- It can be especially helpful if mom is not able to judge her own progress.

- Keep in mind that mirrors do not work for everyone, so be sure to ask mom first and not assume she wants to watch.

see part of your baby's head during contractions. Consider asking the anesthesiologist to lower the epidural dosage if you cannot feel any pressure to push or you are not aware of contractions and you are not making any progress. As long as mom and baby are doing fine, see if you can have more time to push.

If you are not using medication in your labor, you should change your position if the baby's head is not descending. Ideas include hands-knees, sitting on the toilet, and lying on your side.

ZOOM

If you watch a birth video, you might think that you can push your baby out in three contractions. You are watching a film that has been edited, so the sense of time is greatly distorted. The reality is that pushing can take several hours with your first baby.

## Side-lying

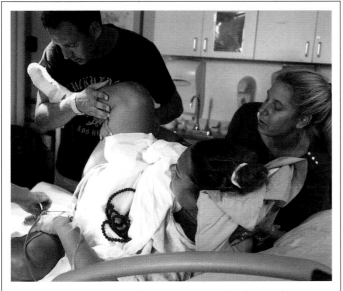

- One of the most versatile positions for pushing is a side-lying position.

- This works well because it allows mom to rest in between her pushes.

- It can also be used to rotate a baby's head from posterior to anterior.

- Pushing in a side-lying position works regardless of whether or not the mother has an epidural.

## Squatting

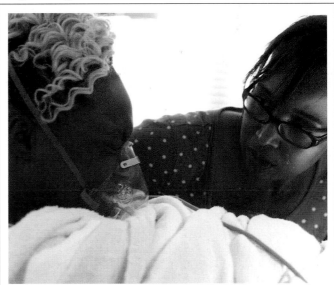

- In some women, squatting can open up the pelvis by as much as 30 percent.

- Check with your place of birth to see if they have a squatting bar attachment that fits over the bed.

- Avoid squatting if your care provider suspects the baby is still in a posterior position.

- You can also use two support people, one on either side of the mother, as she uses a squatting position.

# HIGHS & LOWS

## Mothers may have trouble sleeping in the first 24 hours after birth, even though they are exhausted

Even if your labor was a three-day marathon, chances are high that you will have a surprising amount of energy in the first hours after you give birth. This childbirth "high" is due to the secretion of oxytocin, known as the "love hormone," that reaches its peak immediately after the moment of birth. Having this burst of energy helps to prepare you for the demands

of taking care of your baby, including feeding him or her.

Meanwhile, your body has also been secreting endorphins, natural opiate-like painkillers, during labor. The baby has been releasing its own endorphins, so in the first hour after birth, you and your baby are literally bathed in a sense of warmth, love, and pleasure. Having this first hour to yourselves to

### You May Notice in the First Day:

- you have an immediate "high" right after birth.

- your body will be sore.

- you have trouble turning off your brain.

- you wonder if your birth really happened.

- you begin to bond with your baby.

*Learning about Baby*

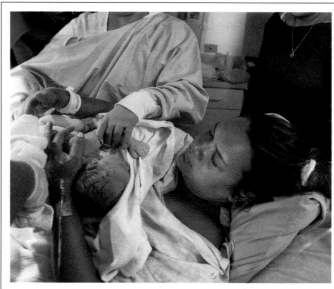

- The first day will give you an opportunity to begin to learn about your baby.

- You might notice your baby's movements are the same ones you have felt for months in your womb.

- You will begin to learn how your baby likes to be held and comforted.

- Your baby will also start responding to your touch, your smell, and your voice.

touch, talk to, and get to know your baby is the perfect way to begin the process of attachment.

Your body will need rest, good nutrition, and possibly pain medication to help you in your physical recovery. If you have swelling or stitches, your labor nurse will often be providing ice packs to reduce pain. As you come down from your "high," sometimes realities of labor play over and over in your mind. Mothers often have a hard time shutting off their brains. However, don't be surprised if in the first twenty-four hours you have to remind yourself that you are now a mother.

In the first twenty-four hours, your uterus will still be contracting in order begin to return to its pre-pregnant size by week six postpartum. These "after-pains" will often occur while you are breast-feeding. If this is your first baby, these after-pains are generally mild, but for second or later babies, the after-pains are more intense. Do not hesitate to ask for pain medication should you need it.

## More Ice Please

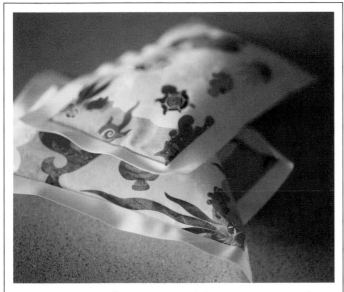

- For some moms, the physical recovery can be a challenging part of the first twenty-four hours.

- Swelling in your pelvic floor will simply add to your pain, so use plenty of ice packs continuously for the first twenty-four hours.

- It is not uncommon to have hemorrhoids after birth, so talk to you care provider about the use of witch hazel pads.

- A warm shower and lots of massage can help to ease your body soreness.

## Processing Your Birth

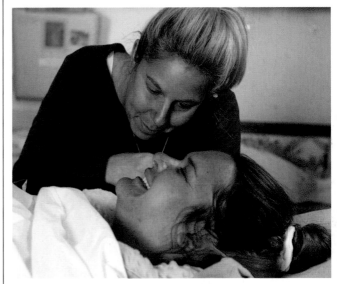

- Part of your recovery involves processing the birth and how it impacted you.

- Mothers have a need to share the events of their birth with as many people as possible.

- Finding the right people who understand you and do not dismiss or minimize events will be important to you.

- One of the benefits of having a birth doula is that she can help you process the highs and lows of your birth experience.

# BABY'S FIRST DAY

Your baby's priorities are to be close to you and to be fed in the first twenty-four hours after birth

As soon as your baby enters the world outside your protective uterus, your care provider will be making sure his airway is clear and that he is kept warm. Research shows that one of the best ways for the baby to regulate his temperature is to be skin-to-skin on his mother.

The more time you spend snuggling up close to your baby in the first twenty-four hours, the better. Your baby will enjoy sharing warmth from your body, hearing your heartbeat, and getting to know your scent. Remember that your voice is already a familiar sound to your baby, so just talking to your baby in soothing tones while you are holding him will often help to comfort him when he is upset.

## What Your Baby Needs

- warmth
- to be held closely by mother or father
- to be breast/bottle-fed
- to be comforted

*Sleep Baby Sleep*

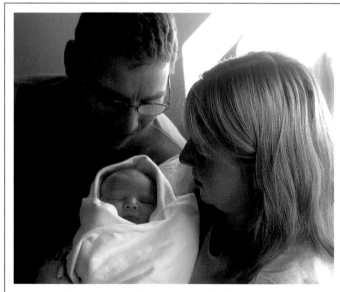

- You might be surprised that your baby is alert and awake for the first few hours after birth.

- After that initial alert time, babies often go into a long period of sleep.

- While this gives you a nice break to begin your recovery, do not let your baby sleep for many hours.

- If your baby sleeps for more than three to four hours straight, it is a good idea to wake her up to be fed.

Any time mother needs a break or is resting, dad can spend time to get to know his baby as well. Fathers' voices will also be a familiar sound to their babies. Mothers should be reminded that fathers will have their own way of bonding with their little one.

If you are breastfeeding, feed your baby as often as possible in the first twenty-four hours to help your milk come in. If you plan to formula-feed your baby, follow the feeding instructions your nurse or care provider gives you.

············· YELLOW ● LIGHT ··············
Research shows that bathing a baby or washing her hands right after birth may interfere with her ability to breastfeed. A similar substance is secreted by both the mother's breast and the amniotic fluid, so bathing removes some of the baby's ability to find her way to her mother's breast. You might request that the bath wait until the following day or until breastfeeding is well established.

## Father and Baby

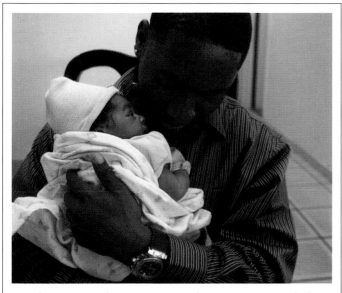

- Fathers are not always instantly confident in caring for their little ones.

- However, very soon they will learn their own ways of relating to their son or daughter.

- Mothers need to allow fathers the space to bond in their unique way with their child.

- In fact, research says that fathers who spend several minutes of "dad and baby" time in the first few hours of life spent more time with their infants at three months of age.

## On Demand

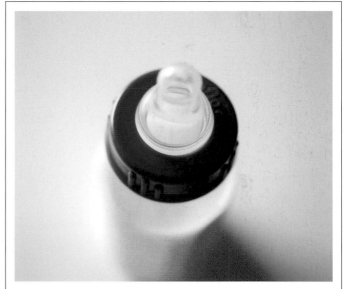

- One of the best ways to encourage your milk to come in sooner is to nurse your baby on demand.

- This requires that you follow the baby's cues and not a schedule or the clock.

- However, if you have a baby that wants to nurse 24/7, your body will need a rest. Offer a pinky finger for a few minutes just to calm baby.

- Then you or dad can wrap baby in a tight swaddle and rock him so that you can get a short break from nursing.

219

# RESTING AFTER BIRTH

## If you are breastfeeding, find out what medication is safe to take for postpartum pain

Whether you are still in your place of birth or already at home, you will undoubtedly be trying to rest and recuperate while trying to take care of all of your baby's needs. If you are in the hospital for a few days, take advantage of the support from your postpartum nurse and lactation consultants. Ask questions about your own self-care and baby care if you are not sure! If you are in pain, find out what medications are safe to take if you are breastfeeding. Getting good pain relief will help you feel more confident in your new role. When you get home, take advantage of help from family and friends.

Part of your recovery involves good nutrition. It is a great idea to stick to your good eating habits from pregnancy.

### Tips for Recovery

- Get help from hospital staff.
- Take pain meds if you need them.
- Recruit help from friends or family at home.
- Sleep when the baby sleeps.
- Hire a postpartum doula.

### Postpartum Medication

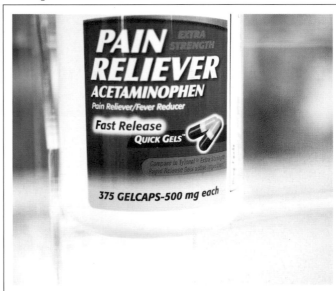

PAIN RELIEVER EXTRA STRENGTH
ACETAMINOPHEN
Pain Reliever/Fever Reducer
Fast Release
QUICK GELS
Compare to Tylenol® Extra Strength Rapid Release Gels active ingredient
375 GELCAPS-500 mg each

- If you have an uncomplicated vaginal birth, you may not need pain medication in your postpartum period.

- Mothers who are experiencing pain should talk to their care providers about appropriate types of pain medication and dosages.

- The most common over-the-counter postpartum medications are acetaminophen, naprosyn, and ibuprofen.

Don't forget that if you are breastfeeding, you will need to add an additional 500 or more calories to your diet before pregnancy, or 200 additional calories to your pregnancy diet. You will likely notice that you are hungrier than ever, and eating in response to that hunger will allow you to add just the right amount of extra calories.

Prioritize your time and energy in the first few days by taking care of yourself and your baby only. Do your best to limit visitors in your first few weeks postpartum. If you are taking good care of yourself, you can better care for your baby.

## Postpartum Diet

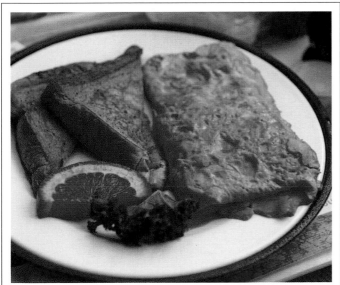

- Make sure you are getting enough dietary iron to replace your blood supply.

- Iron can come from foods such as leafy green vegetables, enriched cereals, and meats.

- Since you may have stitches or discomfort in your pelvic floor, eating plenty of fiber-rich foods is essential.

- You will be highly motivated during the postpartum period to make your first trips to the bathroom a bit easier.

## Sleep When Baby Sleeps

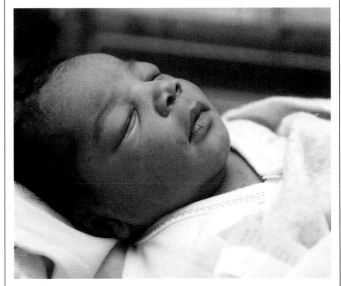

- Your need for sleep will be great in your recovery period.

- The first few days after you give birth, try to get into the habit of sleeping when your baby is sleeping.

- Remember that your baby cannot read the clock, so 2:00 a.m. will be no different to your baby than 2:00 p.m.

# RECOVERING AFTER A CESAREAN

## Moms may find a "football" hold position for breastfeeding is more comfortable after a cesarean

If you are recuperating from a cesarean birth, your early post-partum period will look a bit more challenging. You are likely to spend three to four days at the hospital instead of two days after a vaginal birth. It is common to need stronger pain medication than if you had a vaginal birth.

You will need to adapt your breastfeeding positions after having a cesarean. Sometimes the "cradle hold" position, which places the baby across your chest, may irritate your stitches when you are sitting. You may find that a "football hold," or nursing while on your side, is more comfortable after a cesarean. Staying in the hospital for a longer time means you can take advantage of breastfeeding support.

### What to Expect

- longer stay in hospital
- clear fluids for first day
- stronger pain meds
- help moving around after birth
- need to adjust breastfeeding positions
- limits on stairs and driving

### Post-cesarean Diet

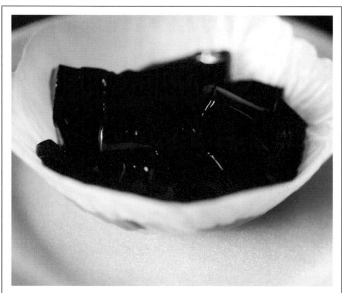

- Regional anesthesia that is required for a cesarean birth will slow the digestive process.

- Because of this sluggishness, if you try to eat solids right away after surgery, you may get sick.

- In the first twelve to twenty-four hours after a cesarean, you will be advised to eat/drink clear fluids such as broth, Jell-O, and clear juices, then slowly progress to solid food.

- After that, you can gradually go back to eating a normal diet.

If you have never had abdominal surgery before your cesarean, it may come as a surprise to recognize how often you use those muscles. Reaching for things, laughing, sneezing, coughing, and rolling over in bed will be uncomfortable for the first few days as you recover from a cesarean. Your nurse will encourage you to get up and walk to the bathroom with her help in the evening or morning after surgery, to help you get back to normal.

## Pain Medications

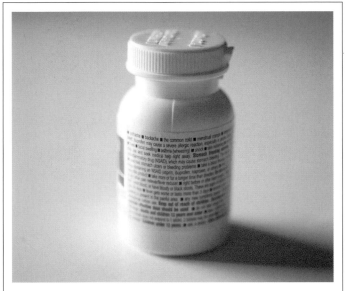

- A cesarean birth is considered to be major abdominal surgery.

- Not only is your recovery longer, but it is likely to be more painful than having a vaginal birth.

- Some mothers find that they need stronger pain medication when healing from surgery.

- A popular post-cesarean pain medication that your care provider may prescribe is Percocet, which is a combination of oxycodone and acetaminophen.

## Other Nursing Positions

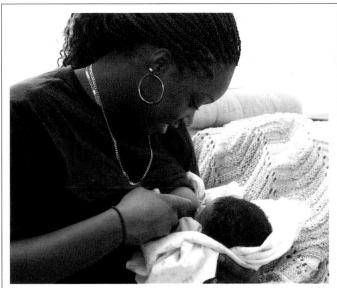

- You might request that your labor nurse or lactation consultant instruct you in the lying-down and football hold positions.

- It is worth the extra time to learn to nurse lying down and with the baby tucked under your arm because they take pressure off your abdominal stitches.

- The lying-down position is also a favorite one among mothers for convenience with nighttime feedings.

- The football hold is also an effective position for a small baby or mothers with larger breasts.

# YOU'RE A MOM!

## Mothers soon learn that there are both joys and challenges to motherhood

Your pregnancy and birth are over. You are now home with your baby and face the difficulties each day brings. For some mothers, the late-night feedings and sleepless nights are one of the hardest things to cope with in the early days. For others, managing symptoms of postpartum mood swings seems to overwhelm them. Undoubtedly you will have days when you think you are not cut out to be a mother. Yet the very next day, you take one look at your baby and you realize that all of the challenges of pregnancy, birth, and postpartum were completely worth it!

One aspect of parenting that cannot be overemphasized is the importance of having good support in your early weeks

### Falling in Love

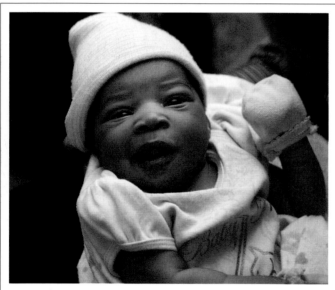

- No matter how many times you hear it, new parents are still surprised by the depth of this amazing love relationship and growing bond that starts between them and their babies.

- While some mothers bond immediately with their babies, it can take others longer to sense that intense connection to their babies.

- Some parents may not feel that "love at first sight" with their babies.

- However, in time, your bond with grow; typically in a few weeks you will sense a bond with your baby.

### Making Mistakes

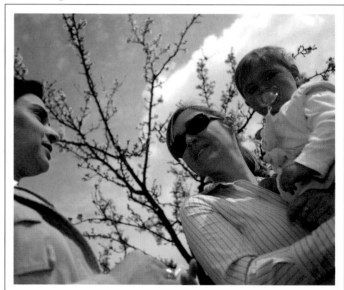

- There is no such thing as a perfect parent. We all get stressed out and lose our tempers. We all do or say things we regret.

- One of the best things about parenthood is that we can learn from our mistakes.

- Why not bounce the situation off another parent to see what advice they can give you to parent your baby more effectively?

- In the end, sometimes the only thing to do is to offer an apology and do things differently the next day.

and months of being a mother. A supportive partner or a good friend with a listening ear who allows you to vent your frustrations from time to time is often all you need.

Remember that your marriage needs reinvestment even when you feel like you barely have enough energy to see straight. Your marriage will go through plenty of its own adjustment during this time. If you find that you are both struggling in your relationship, do not wait to get help.

Congratulations on becoming the best mother and father you can be for your baby.

## Marriage Adjustments

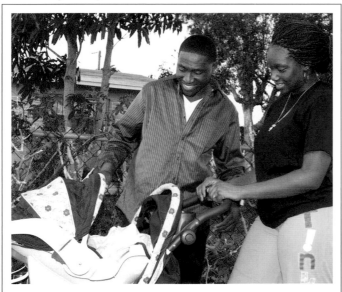

- Bringing a new baby into your life changes the dynamics of the marriage.

- It requires role adjustments, understanding, forgiveness, and self-sacrifice.

- All of these changes happen at a time when you are also struggling with getting enough sleep.

- The key is talking to each other regularly and asking for help to keep your relationship healthy and strong.

## Parenting 101

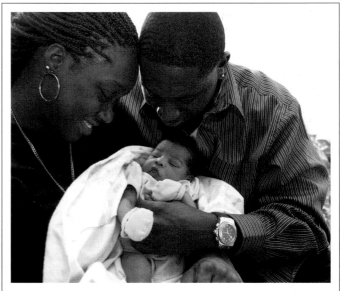

- No single book on parenting holds all of the answers to your parenting questions.

- Nor is any one parenting method the right way to raise every child.

- As you learn more and more what your baby needs, you will grow more confident in your own decision-making.

- You will both discover over time what works with your baby, your lifestyle and your belief system as you strive to be the very best parents you can be.

# RESOURCES

The *Knack Pregnancy Guide* resource directory includes a list of Internet Web sites that provide you with more detailed information, medical research, and articles written by experts in the field, as well as where to find supplies mentioned in this book. While this is not an all-inclusive list, the Web sites highlighted in each section can be an additional resource in your own planning and decision-making. Many of these sites also include helpful tips to guide you each step of the way throughout pregnancy and into the early stages of parenting your baby.

## Chapter 1: Planning

Basal Body Temperature Thermometer:
www.target.com

College Savings Plans:
www.collegesavings.org

Eco-Friendly Baby Furniture and Products:
www.greatgreenbaby.com
www.pristineplanet.com

Inexpensive Ovulation Kits and Pregnancy Tests:
www.accuratepregnancytests.com

Interactive Ovulation Chart (free):
www.fertilityfriend.com

More on Vulvodynia:
www.mayoclinic.com/health/vulvodynia/DS00159

## Chapter 2: Healthy Nutrition

Education Pamphlet on Nutrition During Pregnancy:
www.acog.org/publications/patient_education/bp001.cfm

More Information on Folic Acid:
www.nutramed.com/nutrients/folate.htm

Nutritional Information:
www.nutritiondata.com
www.whfoods.org

Other Information:
www.ncbi.nlm.nih.gov/pubmed/11389286

## Chapter 3: Pregnancy Diet

Healthy Recipes:
www.lowfatlifestyle.com
www.medicinenet.com
www.cookinglight.com

Information on Additives/Preservatives in Foods:
www.naturalpath.com
www.healthyeatingadvisor.com

Organic Foods and Pregnancy:
http://pregnancychildbirth.suite101.com

Slow Cookers:
www.nextag.com
www.target.com

Slow Cooker Recipes:
www.southernfood.about.com
www.slowandsimple.com
www.crockpot.cdkitchen.com

## When to Call Your Care Provider:

- Vaginal bleeding
- Lightheadedness or dizziness
- Headache
- Increased shortness of breath
- Chest pain
- Muscle weakness
- Calf pain
- Uterine contractions
- Decreased movement of the baby
- Leaking vaginal fluid

# Chapter 4: Exercise

Fitness/Birth Balls with Pump:
www.bigfitness.com
www.amazon.com
www.yogadirect.com

More on Diastasis Recti:
www.befitmom.com/abdominal_seperation.html

Pregnancy Exercise Guidelines:
www.acog.org/publications

Strength Training:
www.womenshealthcaretopics.com

Walking Shoes Guidelines:
www.mayoclinic.com/health/walking/HQ00885_D

# Chapter 5: Prenatal Testing

AFP Test:
www.pregnancy.about.com/cs/afp/a/afptesting.htm

Amniocentesis:
www.webmd.com/baby/guide/amniocentesis

Genetic Counseling:
www.marchofdimes.com

NFT Test:
www.babycenter.com/0_nuchal-translucency-screening_118.bc

Ultrasound:
www.americanpregnancy.org/prenataltesting/ultrasound.html

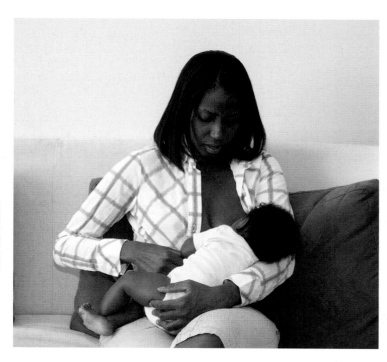

## Chapter 6:
## Select a Provider

Birth Doulas:
www.dona.org

Comparison of Care Providers:
www.transitiontoparenthood.com
www.amazingpregnancy.com

Finding a Perinatologist:
www.ehow.com

More on Childbirth Statistics:
www.childbirthconnection.org

More Questions to Ask:
www.parenting.ivillage.com
www.parentsconnect.com

## Chapter 7: Your Birth Place

Baby-Friendly Hospitals in the U.S.:
www.babyfriendlyusa.org

Birth Centers in the U.S.:
www.birthcenters.org

Questions to Ask:
www.birthing-options.suite101.com
www.childbirthconnection.org
www.pregnancy.about.com

Teaching Hospitals in the U.S.:
www.healthlinksusa.com

## Chapter 8: Childbirth Class

American Academy of Husband-Coached Childbirth (Bradley Method):
www.bradleybirth.com

Birth Works International:
www.birthworks.org

HypnoBirthing:
www.hypnobirthing.com

Lamaze Childbirth:
www.lamaze.org

Other Childbirth Methods:
www.icea.org
www.hypnobabies.com
www.birthingfromwithin.com

# Chapter 9:
# 1st Trimester: Mom

All Natural Prenatal Vitamins:
www.herbalremedies.com
www.naturallydirect.net

Ginger Pops for Morning Sickness:
www.morningsicknesshelp.com

Liquid Prenatal Vitamins:
www.luckyvitamin.com

More on Artificial Sweeteners:
www.medicinenet.com

More on Mercury Levels in Fish:
www.fda.gov/bbs/topics/news/2004/NEW01038.html

More on Soft Cheeses:
www.cfsan.fda.gov/~dms/listeren.html

The Relief Band:
www.amazon.com

# Chapter 10:
# 1st Trimester: Baby

Dr. Peter Nathanielsz and the Prenatal Prescription:
www.pbrc.edu

Fetal Development in the First Trimester:
www.babycenter.com

More on Miscarriage:
www.pregnancyloss.info
www.webmd.com

More on Pregnancy and Relaxation:
www.birthingnaturally.net
www.femail.com.au

Progressive Relaxation Exercises:
www.pregnancy.about.com

# Chapter 11:
# 2nd Trimester: Mom

BMI Calculator:
www.fitpregnancy.com

Finding a Nanny:
www.nanny.com
www.nannies4hire.com

Finding Au Pairs:
www.aupairusa.org
www.aupairinamerica.com

More on Bed Rest:
www.parents.com

More on Day-care Centers:
www.familydoctor.org

Summary of Day-care Options:
www.childcare.about.com

# Chapter 12:
# 2nd Trimester: Baby

AAP Immunization Schedule:
www.cispimmunize.org/IZSchedule_Childhood

AAP Policy Statement on SIDS and Sleep Position/Environment:
http://aappolicy.aappublications.org/cgi/content/abstract/
pediatrics;116/5/1245

Fetal Development Slide Show Month-by-Month:
www.webmd.com/baby/slideshow-fetal-development

Furniture Safety Guidelines:
www.aap.org

More on Co-Sleeping:
www.attachmentparenting.org
www.askdrsears.com

More on Thimerosal:
www.fda.gov/cber/vaccine/thimerosal
www.nationalautismassociation.org

# Chapter 13:
# 3rd Trimester: Mom

Body Pillows:
www.comfortchannel.com
www.shopping.yahoo.com

Comparison of Water Filter Systems:
www.waterfiltercomparisons.com

Insomnia Help:
www.womenshealth.gov
www.pregnancytoday.com

Leg Wedge Pillows:
www.amazon.com
www.makemeheal.com

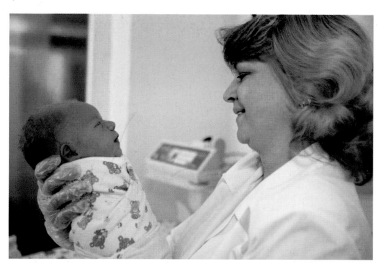

More on Posterior Babies:
www.spinningbabies.com

Natural Massage/Aromatherapy Oils:
www.pristineplanet.com
www.bestmassage.com

Standard Smoke Detectors:
www.homedepot.com

Straps to Anchor Furniture:
www.childsafetystore.com
www.amazon.com

Vocal Smoke Detector:
www.amazon.com

White-noise Machines:
www.naturestapestry.com
www.amazon.com
www.sleepwellbaby.com

# Chapter 14:
# 3rd Trimester: Baby

Baby Name Web Sites:
www.babyhold.com
www.thinkbabynames.com

Baby Shower Favors:
www.mybabyshowerfavors.com

Baby Shower Games:
www.babyshowerstuff.com

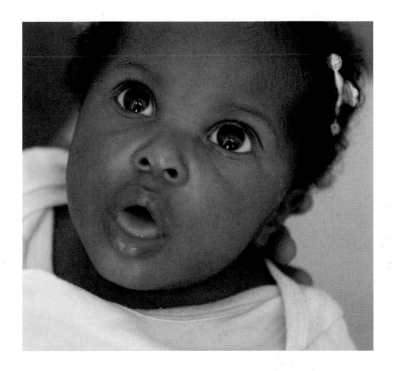

Baby Shower Recipes:
www.bettycrocker.com
www.southernfood.about.com
www.allrecipes.com

Pets and New Baby:
www.hsus.org
www.animalhealthchannel.com

Sibling Adjustment Information:
www.parentingresources.suite101.com

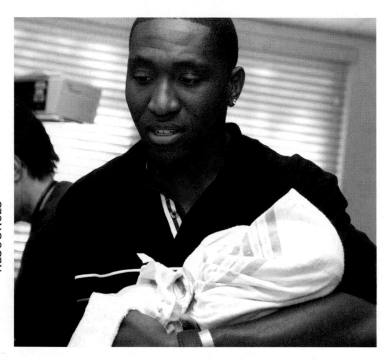

Turning a Breech Baby:
www.midwiferyservices.org
http://pregnancychildbirth.suite101.com/article.cfm/
turning_a_breech_baby

# Chapter 15: Labor & Birth

Energy Bars:
www.kashi.com
www.amazon.com

Kegel Exercise Device:
www.kegelmaster.pro

Make-ahead Meal Recipes:
www.cooks.com
www.lynnescountrykitchen.net

More on Episiotomies:
www.ahrq.gov/consumer/episiotomy.htm
www.mothering.com

Perineal Massage Oil:
www.babybellybotanicals.com
www.nurturecenter.com

# Chapter 16: Birth Plans

Acupressure Points for Labor:
http://pregnancychildbirth.suite101.com/article.cfm/
pressure_points_to_induce_labor

Birth Plan Information:
www.birthingnaturally.net/birthplan/how.html

Comparison of Pain Medications:
www.babies.sutterhealth.org

Interactive Birth Plan:
www.childbirth.org
www.birthplan.com

More on Amniotomy (Breaking the Water):
www.cochrane.org/reviews/en/ab006167.html

More on Birth Positions:
www.givingbirthnaturally.com/birth-positions.html

More on Circumcision:
www.familydoctor.org
www.mayoclinic.com/health/circumcision/PR00040

More on Electronic Fetal Monitoring:
www.babycenter.com

More on Pitocin:
www.massagetoday.com/archives/2006/03/11.html
www.drugs.com/pro/pitocin.html

Pregnancy Loss and Grief Support:
www.babylosskit.com/resources.html
www.nationalshareoffice.com

# Chapter 17: Feeding Your Baby

AAP Guideline on Breastfeeding:
www.aap.org/advocacy/releases/feb05breastfeeding.htm

Baby Bath Accessories:
www.store.babycenter.com

Breast Pumps:
www.worldwidesurgical.com
www.breastpumps.com

Breast Pump Replacement Parts and Storage:
www.momsmaternity.com

Comparison of Human Breast Milk to Formula:
www.askdrsears.com

More on Baby Bathing:
http://pediatrics.about.com/od/newborntips/a/04_bath_baby.htm

More on Infant Formula:
www.healthcastle.com/infant-formula.shtml

More on Pacifiers:
www.mayoclinic.com/health/pacifiers/PR00067

# Chapter 18: Birth: What Is It Like?

Dura*Kold Ice Wraps:
www.amazon.com

Herbal Heat Packs:
www.reliefmart.com
www.healthandbodystore.com

Massage Techniques for Labor:
www.birthingnaturally.net/cn/technique/massage.html

More on Hydrotherapy:
www.expectantmothersguide.com
www3.interscience.wiley.com/journal/77502695/abstract

More on Water Birth:
www.waterbirth.org

# Chapter 19: The First 24 Hours

Baby Swaddling Blankets:
www.thewoombie.com
www.nurturecenter.com

More on Postpartum Depression:
www.mayoclinic.com/health/postpartum-depression/DS00546

Parenting Support:
www.pepsgroup.org
www.kellymom.com
www.parenting.com

Postpartum Doulas:
www.dona.org

Support for Postpartum Depression:
www.postpartum.net

Treatment for Postpartum Depression:
www.helpguide.org/mental/postpartum_depression.htm
http://pregnancychildbirth.suite101.com/article.cfm/
postpartum_depression

Witch Hazel Pads:
www.shopinprivate.com
www.quickmedical.com

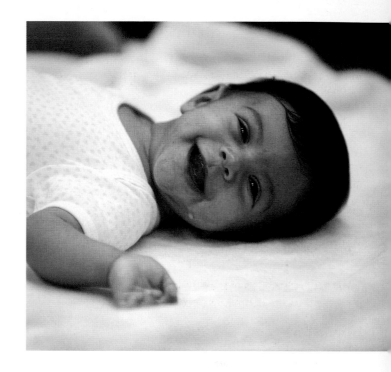

# GLOSSARY

**amniotic fluid:** liquid in the sac that surrounds the baby during pregnancy

**amniotomy (artificial rupture of membranes):** breaking the mother's water using a plastic hook

**antibody:** protein made by the body which destroys other cells such as toxins or bacteria

**after-pains:** contractions of the uterus in the first several days after birth

**areola:** dark area surrounding the nipple of the breast

**basal body temperature:** lowest temperature of healthy person taken as soon as they awaken

**bed rest:** a restriction of the mother's activity, prescribed by some providers for certain pregnancy complications

**birth doula:** a professional support person who offers physical comfort, emotional support, and assistance in finding information before, during and after birth

**breech:** when the baby's head is at the top of the mother's uterus

**Braxton-Hicks contractions:** mild, sporadic practice contractions of the uterus that become more frequent in late pregnancy

**cervix:** lowest and narrowest part of the uterus

**circumcision:** removal of the foreskin of the penis; often done for religious or cultural reasons

**colostrums:** the fluid in the mother's breasts from pregnancy through the first few days of postpartum; rich in antibodies and protein

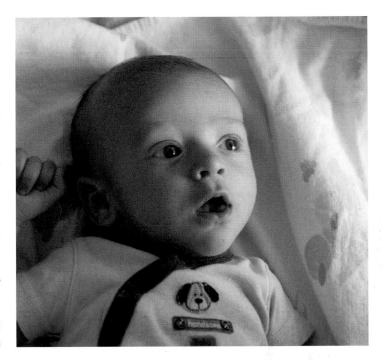

**electronic fetal monitoring:** use of ultrasound to monitor and record the baby's heart rate during labor; methods include continuous or intermittent fetal monitoring

**endometriosis:** a condition in which tissue resembling the uterine lining grows outside the uterus, causing pain, pressure and irregular menstrual periods

**episiotomy:** surgical cut into the mother's perineum during pushing

**forceps:** instruments used to apply traction to the baby's head to assist the mother in pushing

**free-standing birth center:** a facility not attached to a hospital or other medical facility that provides prenatal, birth and immediate postpartum care for the laboring family

**gestational diabetes:** an inability to process carbohydrates that appears during pregnancy

**group B Strep (Streptococcus agalactiae):** a bacteria that is found in 10-35 percent of women often without symptoms for the mother, but can cause infection in the newborn

**hCG (human chorionic gonadotropin):** a hormone produced by cells that form the placenta; it is a marker for pregnancy found in the mother's urine or blood

**high risk:** when pregnancy has an increased possibility of developing complications

**hydrotherapy:** use of water to provide pain relief

**isoflavone:** organic compound that contain estrogen-like qualities; most come from legumes

**jaundice:** when the baby's skin becomes yellowish due to excessive amounts of bilirubin.

**meconium:** dark, sticky, and sterile first stool of the baby

**neural tube defects:** faulty development of the neural tube, which forms the brain and spinal cord

**NICU:** Neonatal Intensive Care Unit; a special nursery in the hospital designed for sick or preterm babies

**nipple confusion:** when baby has difficulty breastfeeding after using a bottle or a pacifier

**nipple stimulation:** stroking, kneading or pumping the breasts in order to start or strengthen contractions

**perineum:** area of tissue between the vagina and the rectum

**perineal massage:** massage done during pregnancy to increase the flexibility of the perineum

**pica:** cravings for non-edible food items during pregnancy such as dirt, starch, or clay

**postpartum doula:** a professional who provides assistance to new parents in breastfeeding, newborn care, postpartum adjustment, and household organization

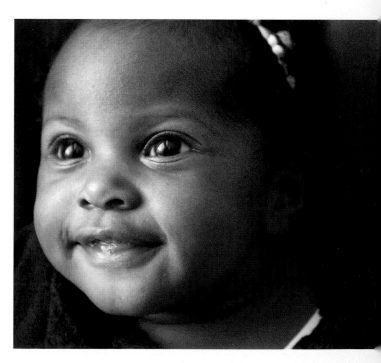

**postpartum mood disorders:** a range of mental health disorders affecting mothers within the first year after giving birth

**pregnancy-induced hypertension (PIH):** elevated blood pressure during pregnancy

**preterm labor:** labor which occurs before thirty-seven weeks of pregnancy

**rooming-in:** when the newborn stays in the same postpartum room with the mother instead of remaining in the nursery

**vernix:** the thick white fatty substance that coats the baby's skin

**vulvodynia:** painful or burning sensation in the vulva, perineum, or labia with touch or pressure

# INDEX